CARNIVORE DIET

Recipes Book

FOR BEGINNER'S SUCCESS

Essential Guide for Beginners with Over 100+ Delectable Recipes, Preparation Tips, Ingredients Lists, and Timings to Revitalize and Energize Your Body for a Healthy Lifestyle

By

PATRICIA T. CONNELL

TABLE OF CONTENTS

In a world saturated with conflicting dietary advice and fad trends promising the elusive path to health and vitality, many find themselves lost in a maze of confusion and frustration. Patricia T. Connell, once a victim of this dietary chaos, knows this struggle all too well.

Like many others, Patricia spent years navigating through countless diets and wellness programs, hoping to find the solution to her health concerns and weight management. From restrictive calorie counting to complicated meal plans, she tried it all, only to end up feeling drained, discouraged, and no closer to her health goals.

But amidst the chaos, Patricia stumbled upon a revelation that would change her life forever – the carnivore diet. Initially met with skepticism and disbelief, she delved deep into the science behind this seemingly radical approach to nutrition.

What she discovered was a simple yet profound truth: our bodies are designed to thrive on a diet rich in animal products, free from the processed foods and additives that plague modern diets.

With renewed hope and determination, Patricia embarked on her carnivore journey, embracing the simplicity and effectiveness of this ancestral way of eating. As she experienced firsthand the transformative power of the carnivore diet – shedding excess weight, experiencing mental clarity, and reclaiming her energy and vitality – Patricia knew she had uncovered a hidden gem that needed to be shared with the world.

And thus, the "Carnivore Diet Recipes Book FOR BEGINNER'S SUCCESS" was born. More than just a collection of recipes, this book is a beacon of hope for those seeking a sustainable, science-backed approach to health and wellness. Drawing from her own experiences and expertise, Patricia has curated over 100 delectable recipes, along with essential preparation tips, ingredient lists, and timings, to guide beginners on their journey to revitalizing and energizing their bodies for a healthy lifestyle.

Join Patricia on this empowering journey as she invites you to discover the transformative potential of the carnivore diet. Say goodbye to confusion and frustration, and embrace a simpler, more natural way of eating that promises to unlock the vibrant health and vitality you've been searching for.

 It's time to take back control of your health and embark on a journey of self-discovery and empowerment with the carnivore diet.

Why this Book?

This book stands out as the ultimate guide for beginners venturing into the world of the carnivore diet. Unlike other diet books that offer generic advice and complex meal plans, "Carnivore Diet Recipes Book FOR BEGINNER'S SUCCESS" provides a unique and comprehensive solution tailored specifically for beginners.

Here's why this book is a must-have:

1. **Expert Guidance**: Authored by Patricia T. Connell, a seasoned advocate and practitioner of the carnivore diet, this book offers expert guidance based on firsthand experience and extensive research. Patricia's journey from confusion to clarity serves as a beacon of hope for beginners, providing them with the confidence and knowledge needed to succeed on their own carnivore journey.

2. **Practical Approach**: This book takes a practical approach to the carnivore diet, focusing on simplicity and effectiveness. With over 100 delectable recipes, preparation tips, ingredient lists, and timings, beginners are equipped with everything they need to kick start their carnivore lifestyle with ease and confidence.

3. **Scientifically Backed**: Backed by scientific evidence and research, the carnivore diet is not just another fad but a sustainable and science-backed approach to health and wellness. This book dives into the science behind the carnivore diet, empowering beginners with a deeper understanding of why this way of eating works and how it can transform their lives.

4. **Personalized Experience**: Unlike one-size-fits-all approaches, this book recognizes the individuality of each beginner and offers a personalized experience. Whether you're a meat lover or new to the carnivore lifestyle, you'll find recipes and tips tailored to your preferences and goals, ensuring a seamless transition to the carnivore way of eating.

5. **Empowering Transformation**: More than just a cookbook, this book is a catalyst for transformation. By embracing the carnivore diet, beginners can expect to experience a wide range of benefits, including weight loss, improved energy levels, mental clarity, and enhanced overall health and vitality. With Patricia's guidance, beginners can unlock their full potential and embark on a journey of self-discovery and empowerment.

In summary, "Carnivore Diet Recipes Book FOR BEGINNER'S SUCCESS" is not just a book – it's a roadmap to a healthier, happier, and more vibrant life. If you're ready to transform your health and embrace the carnivore lifestyle, this book is your ultimate companion on the journey to success.

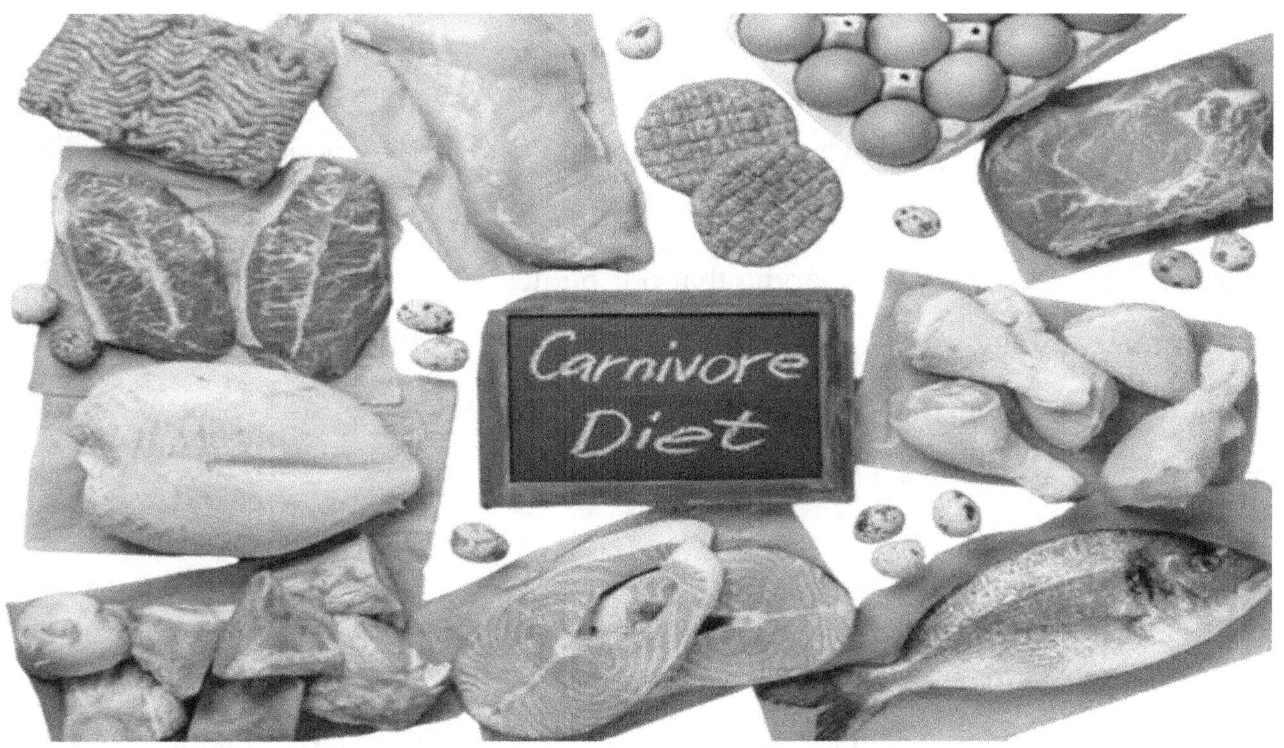

Chapter 1

INTRODUCTION TO THE CARNIVORE DIET

Welcome to the world of the Carnivore Diet, a dietary approach that emphasizes the consumption of animal-based foods while excluding most plant-based foods. In this introductory chapter, we will explore the fundamental principles of the carnivore diet, its potential benefits and challenges, and provide essential tips for beginners to embark on this transformative journey with confidence.

Overview of the Carnivore Diet

The carnivore diet, also known as the zero-carb or all-meat diet, is rooted in the belief that our ancestors primarily subsisted on animal-based foods before the advent of agriculture. Advocates of the carnivore diet argue that our bodies are well-adapted to thrive on a diet rich in animal protein and fat such as meat, fish, eggs, and other animal-based foods, while eliminating or minimizing the consumption of carbohydrates and plant-based foods, including fruits, vegetables, grains, and legumes.

Benefits and Potential Challenges

Proponents of the carnivore diet claim a myriad of potential benefits, including improved weight management, increased energy levels, mental clarity, and reduced inflammation.

Some individuals report relief from various health conditions such as autoimmune disorders, digestive issues, and skin problems.

However, it's essential to acknowledge that the carnivore diet is not without its challenges. Critics raise concerns about potential nutrient deficiencies, particularly in essential vitamins and minerals found in plant-based foods. Additionally, transitioning to a diet devoid of carbohydrates and fiber may cause digestive discomfort for some individuals, at least initially.

Tips for Beginners

Embarking on any new dietary approach can be daunting, especially when navigating uncharted territory like the carnivore diet. As a beginner, it's essential to approach this journey with an open mind and a willingness to learn and adapt. Here are some valuable tips to help you get started on the right foot:

1. **Educate Yourself:** Take the time to research and understand the principles behind the carnivore diet. Familiarize yourself with the allowed foods and potential health benefits to set realistic expectations.

2. **Start Slowly:** Transitioning to a new diet can be challenging, so it's okay to start slowly. Consider gradually reducing the consumption of carbohydrates and plant-based foods while increasing your intake of animal-based foods over time.

3. **Prioritize Quality:** When selecting animal-based foods, prioritize quality over quantity. Opt for grass-fed beef, pasture-raised poultry, wild-caught seafood, and

organically sourced meats whenever possible to maximize nutrient density and minimize exposure to harmful additives.

4. **Listen to Your Body:** Pay attention to how your body responds to the carnivore diet. Monitor changes in energy levels, digestion, mood, and overall well-being. Adjust your dietary approach as needed to optimize your health and vitality.

5. **Stay Hydrated:** Adequate hydration is essential, especially when following a diet high in protein and fat. Drink plenty of water throughout the day to support hydration and optimal bodily functions.

6. **Seek Support:** Joining online communities or seeking guidance from experienced practitioners can provide valuable support and encouragement throughout your carnivore diet journey. Share your experiences, ask questions, and learn from others' experiences to stay motivated and informed.

Remember, embarking on a new dietary approach like the carnivore diet is a journey, not a destination. Be patient with yourself, stay curious, and remain open to learning and adapting along the way. With dedication, mindfulness, and a willingness to explore, you can unlock the potential benefits of the carnivore diet and embark on a path to improved health and vitality.

Chapter 2

GETTING STARTED WITH THE CARNIVORE DIET

Congratulations on taking the first step towards a healthier and more vibrant you by embarking on the carnivore diet journey! In this chapter, I will guide you through the essential steps to get started with the carnivore diet, including setting up your kitchen for success, understanding carnivore-approved foods, and mastering the basics of meal planning, I've got you covered.

Setting up Your Kitchen for Success

The foundation of success on the carnivore diet begins with your kitchen. Creating an environment that supports your dietary goals is key to making the transition smooth and enjoyable. Here are some tips to set up your kitchen for success:

1. **Stock up on carnivore-approved foods:** Fill your pantry and refrigerator with a variety of animal-based foods such as beef, poultry, pork, lamb, seafood, and organ meats. Opt for high-quality, grass-fed, and pasture-raised options whenever possible to maximize nutrient density and flavor. Consider purchasing in bulk to save money and ensure a steady supply of nutritious ingredients.

2. **Eliminate non-carnivore foods:** Remove non-carnivore foods such as grains, legumes, fruits, vegetables, and processed foods from your kitchen to avoid temptation and stay focused on your dietary goals.

3. **Invest in kitchen essentials:** Equip your kitchen with essential tools and equipment for preparing carnivore-friendly meals. This may include a quality chef's knife, cutting board, cast-iron skillet, roasting pan, and meat thermometer.

Investing in quality cooking equipment is essential for making the carnivore diet an enjoyable and sustainable lifestyle choice. Here are additional tips to enhance your kitchen setup for success:

1. **Sharp Knives:** A set of sharp knives is indispensable for preparing meat and other carnivore-approved foods with precision and ease. Invest in high-quality chef's knives, boning knives, and utility knives to handle various cutting tasks efficiently.

2. **Meat Thermometer:** Ensure perfectly cooked meats every time by investing in a reliable meat thermometer. This tool helps you monitor internal temperatures accurately, preventing overcooking or undercooking and ensuring food safety.

3. **Food Storage Containers:** Keep your carnivore-approved foods fresh and organized by investing in a variety of food storage containers. Opt for durable containers that are freezer-safe, microwave-safe, and dishwasher-safe for convenient meal prep and storage.

4. **Quality Cookware:** Choose cookware made from high-quality materials such as stainless steel, cast iron, or enameled cast iron for durability and even heat distribution. Invest in a variety of pots, pans, and baking dishes to accommodate different cooking methods and recipes.

5. **Kitchen Scale:** Achieve precise portion control and accurate measurements by using a kitchen scale. This tool is particularly useful for tracking your protein intake and ensuring consistent results in your carnivore cooking endeavors.

6. **Kitchen Gadgets:** Consider adding useful kitchen gadgets to your arsenal, such as a meat tenderizer, meat grinder, or vacuum sealer, to expand your culinary repertoire and enhance your carnivore cooking experience.

7. **Spices and Seasonings:** While the carnivore diet primarily focuses on animal-based foods, incorporating herbs, spices, and seasonings can add depth and flavor to your meals. Stock up on carnivore-friendly spices such as salt, pepper, garlic powder, and dried herbs to enhance the taste of your dishes.

By equipping your kitchen with the right tools and essentials, you'll create a supportive environment that fosters success on the carnivore diet. With a well-stocked kitchen and quality cooking equipment at your disposal, you'll be ready to embark on a journey of delicious and nutritious carnivore cooking adventures.

Understanding Carnivore-Approved Foods

On the carnivore diet, the primary focus is on consuming animal-based foods while eliminating or minimizing plant-based foods. Here's a breakdown of carnivore-approved foods:

1. **Meat:** Beef, poultry, pork, lamb, venison, bison, and other types of animal meat are staples of the carnivore diet. Opt for fatty cuts of meat and include a variety of cuts to keep your meals interesting.

2. **Seafood:** Fish, shellfish, and other types of seafood are excellent sources of protein and essential nutrients on the carnivore diet. Include a variety of seafood options in your diet to reap the benefits of different nutrients.

3. **Organ meats:** Liver, heart, kidney, and other organ meats are nutrient powerhouses rich in vitamins, minerals, and essential nutrients. Don't shy away from incorporating organ meats into your diet for maximum nutritional benefits.

4. **Eggs:** Include eggs in your diet as a versatile and nutritious source of protein and fat. Choose pastured or omega-3-enriched eggs for added nutritional benefits.

5. **Dairy (optional):** Some individuals on the carnivore diet choose to include dairy products such as cheese, butter, and heavy cream.

However, it's essential to monitor your body's response to dairy and choose high-quality, full-fat options. In addition to the core carnivore-approved foods mentioned above, it's important to understand the nuances of the carnivore diet and how certain foods may impact your body. Here's a deeper dive into carnivore-approved foods and considerations for optimal success:

1. **Meat**: When selecting meats, prioritize quality and diversity. Opt for grass-fed beef, pasture-raised poultry, and wild-caught game meats whenever possible. These options tend to be higher in essential nutrients such as omega-3 fatty acids and contain fewer harmful additives and hormones compared to conventionally raised meats.

2. **Seafood**: Fatty fish like salmon, mackerel, and sardines are excellent choices due to their high omega-3 content, which supports heart health and brain function. When choosing shellfish, opt for varieties low in mercury, such as shrimp, crab, and scallops, to minimize potential health risks.

3. **Organ Meats**: Organ meats are nutritional powerhouses packed with vitamins, minerals, and essential nutrients. Liver, in particular, is a nutrient-dense superfood, rich in vitamin A, B vitamins, iron, and copper. Incorporating a variety of organ meats like heart, kidney, and spleen ensures a well-rounded nutrient profile and supports overall health.

4. **Eggs**: Eggs are a versatile and nutritious addition to the carnivore diet, providing high-quality protein, healthy fats, and essential vitamins and minerals. Opt for pastured or omega-3-enriched eggs whenever possible, as they contain higher levels of beneficial nutrients compared to conventional eggs.

5. **Dairy (optional)**: While dairy products like cheese, butter, and heavy cream are technically carnivore-approved, they may not be well-tolerated by everyone.

Some individuals may experience digestive issues or inflammation in response to dairy consumption, especially if they have lactose intolerance or sensitivities to dairy proteins. If you choose to include dairy in your carnivore diet, opt for high-quality, full-fat options and monitor your body's response closely.

It's essential to listen to your body and pay attention to how different foods impact your health and well-being on the carnivore diet. While these carnivore-approved foods form the foundation of your diet, individual tolerance and preferences may vary. Experiment with different foods, observe how your body responds, and adjust your dietary choices accordingly to optimize your carnivore experience.

Meal Planning Basics

Effective meal planning is essential for success on the carnivore diet. Here are some basic principles to keep in mind when planning your carnivore meals:

1. **Prioritize protein:** Protein should be the centerpiece of your meals on the carnivore diet. Aim to include a generous portion of protein with each meal such as steak, chicken thighs, or salmon fillets to support muscle growth, repair, and overall health.

2. **Include healthy fats:** Add healthy fats to your meals to increase satiety and provide essential nutrients. Opt for animal fats such as tallow, lard, or duck fat, as well as olive oil, avocado oil, and coconut oil.

3. **Keep it simple:** Embrace simplicity when planning your carnivore meals. Focus on high-quality animal-based foods and minimal seasoning to let the natural flavors shine.

4. **Plan ahead:** Take time to plan your meals for the week ahead to ensure you have everything you need on hand. Batch cooking and meal prep can be valuable strategies to save time and streamline your carnivore meal preparation process.

When it comes to meal planning on the carnivore diet, simplicity and nutrient density are key. Here are additional tips to help you create balanced and satisfying carnivore-friendly meals:

1 **Include a variety of animal-based foods**: While prioritizing protein is important, don't forget to vary your sources of animal-based foods to ensure you're getting a wide range of nutrients. Incorporate a mix of red meats, poultry, seafood, and organ meats into your meal rotation to reap the benefits of different nutrient profiles.

2 **Explore different cooking methods**: Experiment with various cooking methods to add variety and flavor to your meals. Whether you're grilling, roasting, pan-searing, or slow-cooking, each method can impart unique textures and tastes to your carnivore dishes.

3 **Embrace seasonings and spices**: While the carnivore diet typically emphasizes minimal seasoning, you can still add flavor to your meals with herbs, spices, and

seasonings that are compatible with the diet. Stick to simple options like salt, pepper, garlic powder, and dried herbs to enhance the natural flavors of your meat without detracting from its nutrient density.

4. **Incorporate bone broth**: Bone broth is a nourishing and versatile addition to the carnivore diet. Rich in collagen, amino acids, and minerals, bone broth can be enjoyed as a warm beverage or used as a base for soups and stews to add depth of flavor and nutritional benefits to your meals.

5. **Consider intermittent fasting**: Many individuals on the carnivore diet find success with intermittent fasting, which involves cycling between periods of eating and fasting. By incorporating intermittent fasting into your meal planning strategy, you can optimize fat-burning, promote metabolic flexibility, and enhance overall health and vitality.

6. **Plan ahead for convenience**: To streamline meal preparation and stay on track with your carnivore diet goals, consider batch cooking and meal prepping ahead of time. Prepare large batches of carnivore-friendly dishes and portion them out into individual servings for easy grab-and-go meals throughout the week.

7. **Stay hydrated**: Hydration is essential for overall health and well-being, especially on a low-carb, high-protein diet like the carnivore diet. Make sure to drink plenty of water throughout the day to stay hydrated and support optimal bodily functions.

By incorporating these meal planning basics into your carnivore diet routine, you can enjoy delicious, nutrient-dense meals that support your health and well-being while staying true to the principles of the carnivore lifestyle. Experiment with different foods, cooking methods, and meal timing to find what works best for you and your individual needs.

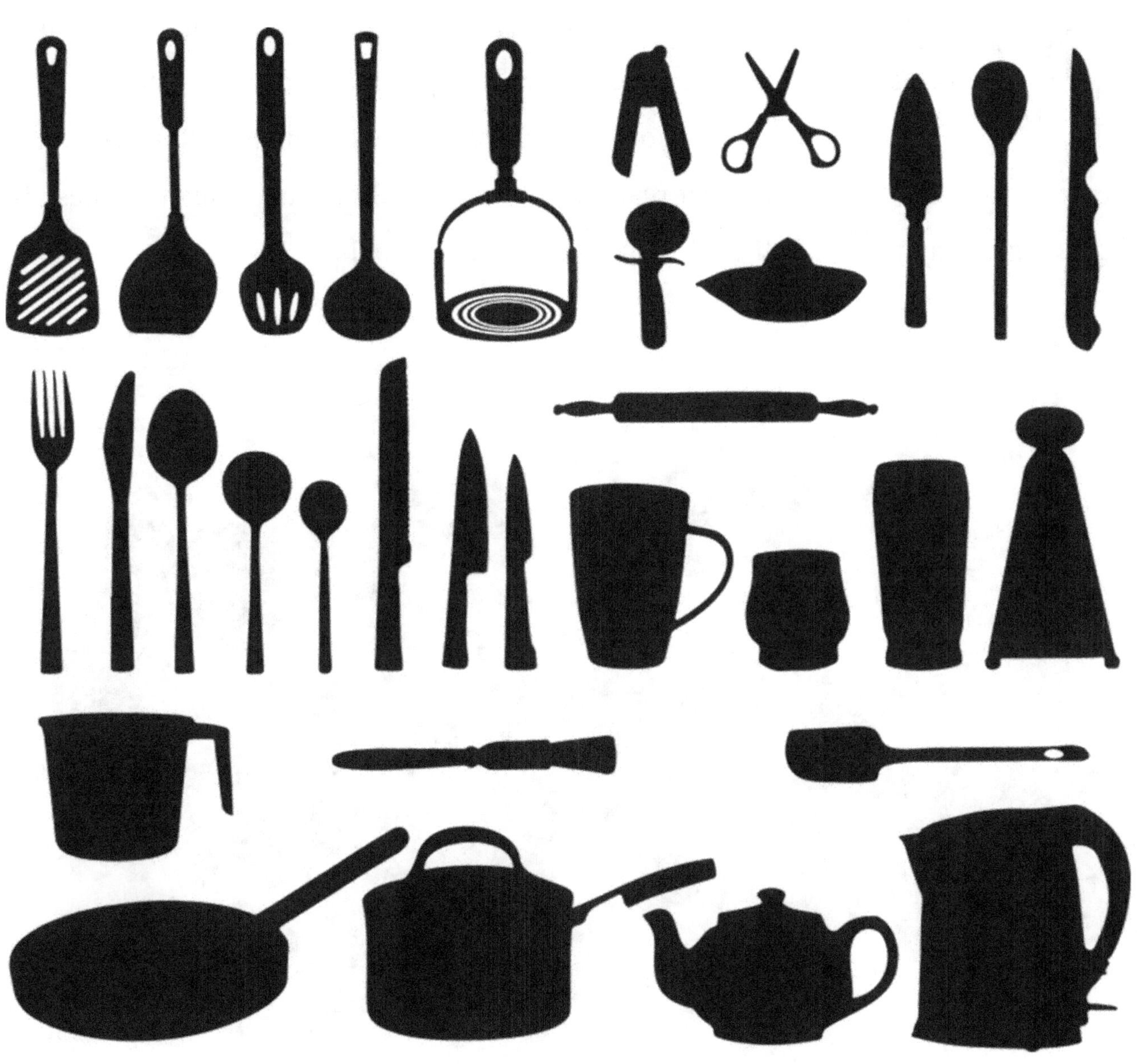

Chapter 3

BEEF DELIGHTS

Welcome to the carnivore culinary journey with a spotlight on the king of meats – beef. In this chapter, we'll explore a variety of delectable beef recipes that not only showcase the versatility of this meat but also cater to different tastes and preferences. Get ready to savor the richness and flavor of these beef delights while staying true to the principles of the carnivore diet.

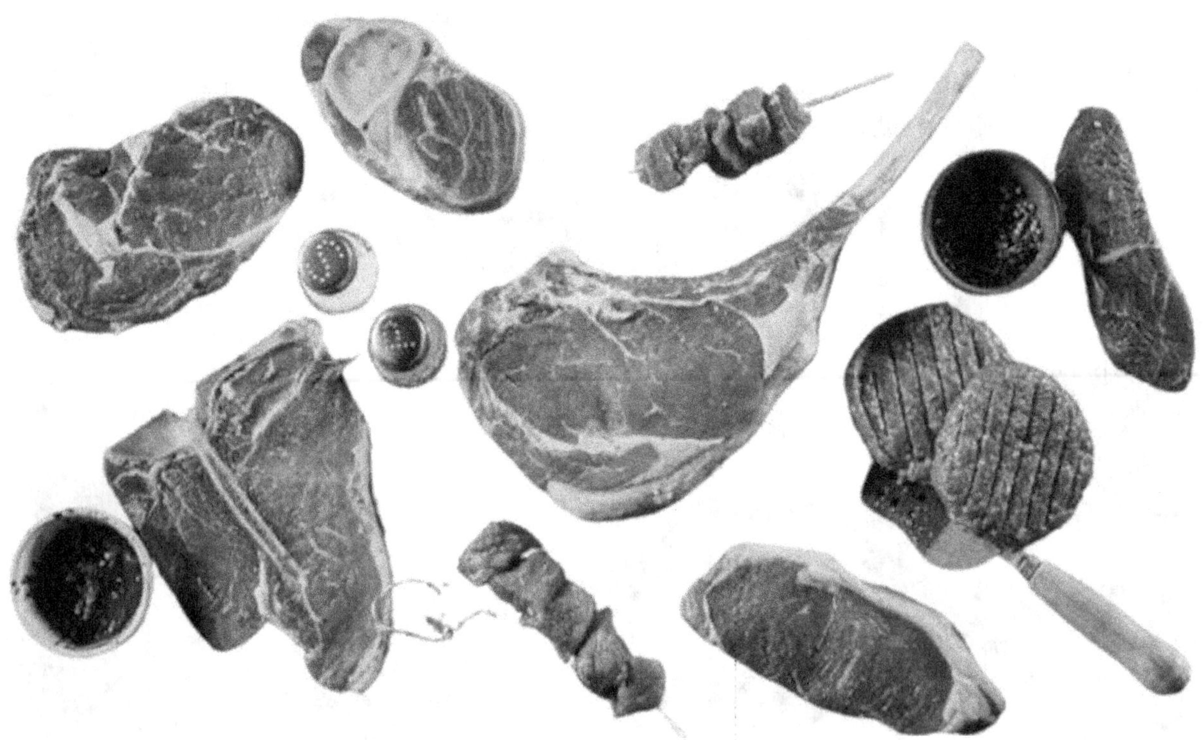

Ribeye Steak with Garlic Butter

Indulge in the rich, buttery goodness of a perfectly seared ribeye steak topped with savory garlic butter. This classic carnivore favorite is sure to satisfy your cravings for juicy, tender beef.

Ingredients:

2 Ribeye steaks (about 1 inch thick)

Salt and black pepper, to taste

2 tablespoons unsalted butter

2 cloves garlic, minced

Fresh parsley, chopped (optional, for garnish)

Step by step Instructions:

1. **Prepare the steaks:** Remove the ribeye steaks from the refrigerator and let them sit at room temperature for about 30 minutes to ensure even cooking.

2. **Season the steaks:** Season both sides of each steak generously with salt and black pepper. This will enhance the flavor of the meat.

3. **Preheat the skillet:** Heat a skillet (preferably cast iron) over medium-high heat until hot. You want the skillet to be hot enough to create a nice sear on the steaks.

4. **Sear the steaks:** Once the skillet is hot, carefully place the seasoned ribeye steaks in the skillet. Cook for about 4-5 minutes on each side for medium-rare, or adjust the cooking time according to your desired level of doneness.

5. **Add the garlic butter:** While the steaks are cooking, melt the unsalted butter in a small saucepan over medium heat. Add the minced garlic to the melted butter and cook for 1-2 minutes, until fragrant.

6. **Baste the steaks:** Once the ribeye steaks are cooked to your liking, remove them from the skillet and transfer them to a plate. Immediately pour the garlic butter over the steaks, using a spoon to baste them with the flavorful butter.

7. **Rest the steaks:** Allow the ribeye steaks to rest for a few minutes before serving. This allows the juices to redistribute throughout the meat, ensuring a juicy and tender steak.

8. **Garnish and serve:** Optional: Sprinkle freshly chopped parsley over the steaks for a pop of color and added flavor. Serve the Ribeye Steak with Garlic Butter hot and enjoy!

Note: Remember to adjust cooking times based on the thickness of your steaks and your desired level of doneness.

Use a meat thermometer to ensure the internal temperature reaches your preferred level of doneness (around 130°F for medium-rare). Enjoy your delicious, juicy Ribeye Steaks with Garlic Butter!

Beef Liver Pâté

Elevate your carnivore cuisine with this luxurious beef liver pâté. Packed with essential nutrients like vitamin A, iron, and B vitamins, this decadent spread is as delicious as it is nutritious.

Ingredients:

1 lb. beef liver, cleaned and trimmed

1 onion, finely chopped

2 cloves garlic, minced

4 tablespoons unsalted butter

1/4 cup heavy cream

1 tablespoon fresh thyme leaves (optional)

Salt and black pepper, to taste

Step by Step Instructions:

1. **Prepare the beef liver:** Rinse the beef liver under cold water and pat it dry with paper towels. Trim any visible connective tissue or membranes from the liver. Cut the liver into small, evenly sized pieces for easier cooking.

2. **Sauté the onions and garlic:** In a skillet, melt 2 tablespoons of unsalted butter over medium heat. Add the finely chopped onion and minced garlic to the skillet. Cook until the onions are soft and translucent, about 5-7 minutes.

3. **Cook the beef liver:** In the same skillet, increase the heat to medium-high. Add the remaining 2 tablespoons of unsalted butter to the skillet. Once melted, add the beef liver pieces to the skillet. Cook the liver until it is browned on the outside but still slightly pink on the inside, about 2-3 minutes per side. Be careful not to overcook the liver, as it can become tough and dry.

4. **Blend the liver mixture:** Transfer the cooked liver, onions, and garlic to a food processor or blender. Add the heavy cream and fresh thyme leaves (if using) to the mixture. Season with salt and black pepper to taste.

5. **Blend until smooth:** Blend the liver mixture until it is smooth and creamy, scraping down the sides of the food processor or blender as needed. If the pâté is too thick, you can add additional heavy cream, one tablespoon at a time, until you reach your desired consistency.

6. **Adjust seasoning:** Taste the pâté and adjust the seasoning as needed, adding more salt and pepper if desired.

7. **Chill and serve:** Transfer the beef liver pâté to a serving dish or ramekins. Cover the pâté with plastic wrap and refrigerate for at least 1-2 hours to allow the flavors to meld together and the pâté to firm up.

8. **Garnish and serve:** Before serving, garnish the beef liver pâté with fresh thyme leaves or a sprinkle of black pepper, if desired. Serve the pâté with carnivore-friendly crackers, vegetable sticks, or enjoy it on its own as a delicious and nutrient-rich spread.

Note: Beef liver pâté can be stored in an airtight container in the refrigerator for up to 1 week. Make sure to cover the pâté with a thin layer of melted butter to help preserve its freshness. Enjoy this luxurious and nutrient-packed Beef Liver Pâté as a tasty addition to your carnivore cuisine!

Beef Jerky

Satisfy your snack cravings with homemade beef jerky, a portable and protein-packed treat that's perfect for on-the-go carnivores. With just a few simple ingredients and a dehydrator, you can enjoy flavorful and satisfying beef jerky anytime, anywhere.

Ingredients:

- 1 lb. beef (preferably lean cuts like flank steak or sirloin)

- 1/4 cup soy sauce or coconut amines (for a gluten-free option)

- 2 tablespoons Worcestershire sauce

- 1 tablespoon honey or maple syrup (optional, for sweetness)

- 1 teaspoon garlic powder

- 1 teaspoon onion powder

- 1/2 teaspoon black pepper

- 1/2 teaspoon smoked paprika (optional, for added flavor)

- 1/4 teaspoon cayenne pepper (optional, for heat)

Step by Step Instructions:

Prepare the beef: Trim any excess fat from the beef and slice it into thin strips, about 1/4 inch thick. For easier slicing, you can partially freeze the beef for about 30 minutes before cutting.

1. **Marinate the beef:** In a bowl, combine the soy sauce (or coconut amines), Worcestershire sauce, honey or maple syrup (if using), garlic powder, onion powder, black pepper, smoked paprika (if using), and cayenne pepper (if using). Stir until well combined.

2. **Marinate the beef strips:** Place the beef strips in a shallow dish or resalable plastic bag. Pour the marinade over the beef, making sure it is evenly coated. Cover the dish or seal the bag, and refrigerate for at least 4 hours, or preferably overnight, to allow the flavors to penetrate the meat.

3. **Preheat the dehydrator:** If using a dehydrator, preheat it to 160°F (or follow the manufacturer's instructions). If using an oven, preheat it to the lowest setting (usually around 170°F).

4. **Prepare the drying racks:** If using a dehydrator, arrange the marinated beef strips in a single layer on the drying racks, leaving space between each strip for air circulation. If using an oven, place a wire rack on top of a baking sheet and arrange the beef strips on the wire rack.

5. **Dehydrate the beef:** Place the beef strips in the dehydrator or oven and allow them to dry for 4-6 hours, or until they are dried to your desired level of chewiness. If using a dehydrator, rotate the drying racks halfway through the drying process for even drying.

6. **Check for doneness:** To check if the beef jerky is done, remove a piece from the dehydrator or oven and allow it to cool for a few minutes. The jerky should be dry to the touch and slightly pliable, but not brittle.

7. **Cool and store:** Once the beef jerky is done, remove it from the dehydrator or oven and allow it to cool completely. Pat any excess oil off the jerky with paper towels. Transfer the beef jerky to an airtight container or resalable plastic bags and store it in a cool, dry place.

Enjoy your homemade Beef Jerky as a delicious and protein-packed snack that's perfect for fueling your on-the-go adventures!

Adjust the seasonings to suit your taste preferences, and experiment with different marinades for endless flavor possibilities.

Beef Bone Marrow Roasted with Salt

Delight your senses with the rich, buttery flavor of roasted beef bone marrow sprinkled with a touch of salt. This nutrient-dense delicacy is a decadent addition to any carnivore meal.

Ingredients:

- Beef marrow bones (sliced lengthwise)
- Coarse sea salt

Step by Step Instructions:

1   **Prepare the beef marrow bones:** Preheat your oven to 425°F (220°C). Place the sliced beef marrow bones on a baking sheet lined with parchment paper or aluminum foil, cut side up.

2   **Score the marrow:** Using a sharp knife, carefully score the surface of the marrow in a crisscross pattern. This will help the salt penetrate and enhance the flavor of the marrow during roasting.

3   **Season with salt:** Sprinkle a generous amount of coarse sea salt evenly over the surface of the marrow bones. The salt will not only add flavor but also help draw out excess moisture from the marrow during roasting.

4   **Roast the marrow bones:** Place the baking sheet with the seasoned marrow bones in the preheated oven. Roast for about 15-20 minutes, or until the marrow is soft and easily scoop able with a spoon. The edges of the bones may start to brown slightly, which is normal and adds flavor.

5   **Serve hot:** Remove the roasted beef marrow bones from the oven and let them cool for a few minutes. Serve the marrow hot, directly from the bones, with crusty bread or carnivore-friendly crackers for spreading.

6   **Enjoy:** Use a small spoon to scoop out the softened marrow from the bones and spread it onto your preferred accompaniment. Savor the rich, buttery flavor of the roasted beef bone marrow sprinkled with salt.

7   **Optional garnish:** For added flavor and freshness, you can garnish the roasted beef bone marrow with chopped fresh herbs, such as parsley or chives, before serving.

8   **Storage:** If you have leftover roasted beef bone marrow, you can store it in an airtight container in the refrigerator for up to 2-3 days. Simply reheat it gently in the oven or microwave before serving.

Indulge in this nutrient-dense delicacy of Beef Bone Marrow Roasted with Salt as a decadent addition to your carnivore meal. The rich, buttery flavor and melt-in-your-mouth texture will delight your senses and elevate your dining experience.

Beef Heart Skewers

Fire up the grill and savor the bold, beefy flavor of beef heart skewers. High in protein and rich in nutrients like iron and B vitamins, beef heart is a delicious and underrated cut that deserves a place on your carnivore menu.

Ingredients:

- 1 beef heart
- Wooden or metal skewers
- Salt and black pepper, to taste
- Olive oil (optional, for brushing)

Step by Step Instructions:

1 **Prepare the beef heart:** Rinse the beef heart under cold water and pat it dry with paper towels. Trim off any excess fat or connective tissue from the beef heart. Cut the beef heart into cubes, about 1 inch in size, for skewering.

2 **Pre-soak the skewers:** If using wooden skewers, pre-soak them in water for at least 30 minutes to prevent them from burning on the grill.

3 **Season the beef heart:** Season the beef heart cubes generously with salt and black pepper, to taste. You can also add additional seasonings or marinade if desired, such as garlic powder, onion powder, or your favorite carnivore-friendly seasoning blend.

4 **Skewer the beef heart:** Thread the seasoned beef heart cubes onto the skewers, leaving a small space between each cube to ensure even cooking. If using metal skewers, make sure to leave enough room at the top and bottom of each skewer for handling.

5 **Preheat the grill:** Preheat your grill to medium-high heat (around 375-400°F) and lightly oil the grates to prevent sticking.

6 **Grill the skewers:** Place the beef heart skewers on the preheated grill, arranging them in a single layer. Grill the skewers for about 3-4 minutes on each side, or until the beef heart is cooked to your desired level of doneness and has nice grill marks.

7 **Optional: Brush with olive oil:** If desired, you can brush the beef heart skewers with olive oil during grilling to help enhance flavor and prevent them from drying out.

8 **Serve hot:** Once the beef heart skewers are cooked to perfection, remove them from the grill and transfer them to a serving platter. Serve the skewers hot and enjoy the bold, beefy flavor of this nutrient-rich carnivore delicacy!

Beef heart skewers make a delicious and nutrient-packed addition to any carnivore meal.

Experiment with different seasonings and marinades to customize the flavor to your liking, and enjoy the rich, beefy goodness of this underrated cut.

Beef Short Ribs Slow-Cooked in Bone Broth

Fall in love with the melt-in-your-mouth tenderness of slow-cooked beef short ribs simmered in savory bone broth. This comforting and hearty dish is perfect for cozy carnivore dinners.

Ingredients:

- 2 lbs. beef short ribs
- 4 cups beef bone broth
- 1 onion, chopped
- 3 cloves garlic, minced
- 2 carrots, chopped
- 2 celery stalks, chopped
- 2 tablespoons tomato paste
- 1 tablespoon Worcestershire sauce
- 1 teaspoon dried thyme
- 1 teaspoon dried rosemary
- Salt and black pepper, to taste
- Fresh parsley, chopped (for garnish)

Step by Step Instructions:

1 **Prepare the short ribs:** Season the beef short ribs generously with salt and black pepper on all sides.

2 **Sear the short ribs:** Heat a large skillet or Dutch oven over medium-high heat. Once hot, add the beef short ribs to the skillet and sear them on all sides until browned, about 3-4 minutes per side. Remove the short ribs from the skillet and set aside.

3 **Prepare the slow cooker:** Place the chopped onion, minced garlic, chopped carrots, and chopped celery in the bottom of a slow cooker.

4 **Add the short ribs:** Arrange the seared beef short ribs on top of the vegetables in the slow cooker.

5 **Make the sauce:** In a small bowl, whisk together the beef bone broth, tomato paste, Worcestershire sauce, dried thyme, and dried rosemary until well combined. Pour the sauce over the beef short ribs and vegetables in the slow cooker.

6 **Cook low and slow:** Cover the slow cooker with the lid and cook the beef short ribs on low heat for 6-8 hours, or until the meat is tender and falls off the bone.

7 **Skim off excess fat (optional):** Once the beef short ribs are cooked, you can skim off any excess fat from the surface of the cooking liquid using a spoon if desired.

8 **Serve:** Remove the beef short ribs from the slow cooker and transfer them to a serving platter. Garnish with freshly chopped parsley for a pop of color and flavor.

9 **Enjoy:** Serve the Beef Short Ribs Slow-Cooked in Bone Broth hot, alongside your favorite side dishes or vegetables, and enjoy the melt-in-your-mouth tenderness and savory flavor of this comforting carnivore dish.

This hearty and comforting dish is perfect for cozy carnivore dinners and is sure to become a favorite in your carnivore meal rotation. Enjoy!

Beef Tongue Tacos with Lettuce Wraps

Put a carnivore twist on taco night with tender beef tongue wrapped in crisp lettuce leaves. Packed with flavor and protein, these lettuce wraps are a refreshing and satisfying alternative to traditional tacos.

Ingredients:

- 1 beef tongue (about 2-3 lbs.)
- 1 onion, quartered
- 3 cloves garlic, smashed
- 2 bay leaves
- 1 teaspoon whole black peppercorns
- Salt, to taste

- Iceberg lettuce leaves (for wrapping)
- Optional toppings: diced tomatoes, diced onions, sliced jalapenos, avocado slices, cilantro leaves, lime wedges

Step by Step Instructions:

1 **Prepare the beef tongue:** Rinse the beef tongue under cold water and place it in a large pot. Add the quartered onion, smashed garlic cloves, bay leaves, whole black peppercorns, and a generous pinch of salt to the pot.

2 **Cook the beef tongue:** Fill the pot with enough water to cover the beef tongue completely. Bring the water to a boil over high heat, then reduce the heat to low and let the tongue simmer, partially covered, for about 3-4 hours or until tender. You can also use a pressure cooker for faster cooking time (about 60-90 minutes).

3 **Cool and peel the tongue:** Once the beef tongue is tender, remove it from the pot and let it cool slightly until it's safe to handle. Use a sharp knife to peel off the tough outer skin of the tongue. Discard the skin and any excess fat.

4 **Slice the tongue:** Slice the beef tongue thinly against the grain to ensure tenderness and easy chewing.

5 **Prepare the lettuce wraps:** Wash and dry the iceberg lettuce leaves. Arrange them on a serving platter to use as taco shells for your beef tongue filling.

6   **Assemble the tacos:** Place a few slices of beef tongue onto each lettuce leaf. Top with your choice of optional toppings, such as diced tomatoes, diced onions, sliced jalapenos, avocado slices, cilantro leaves, and a squeeze of lime juice.

7   **Serve:** Arrange the Beef Tongue Tacos with Lettuce Wraps on a platter and serve immediately. Enjoy the refreshing crunch of the lettuce wraps paired with the tender and flavorful beef tongue filling.

8   **Optional: Sauce or dressing:** You can also serve these tacos with a drizzle of your favorite sauce or dressing, such as salsa Verde, hot sauce, or a creamy cilantro lime dressing, for added flavor.

These Beef Tongue Tacos with Lettuce Wraps are a delicious and satisfying twist on traditional tacos, perfect for a refreshing and protein-packed meal. Enjoy!

Each of these beef delights offers a unique culinary experience while staying true to the principles of the carnivore diet. From succulent steaks to savory stews, these recipes showcase the versatility and deliciousness of beef, making it easy and enjoyable to thrive on the carnivore lifestyle.

POULTRY PLEASURES

Delight your taste buds with a variety of poultry-based carnivore dishes that are both flavorful and satisfying. From succulent chicken thighs to savory turkey meatballs, these recipes will add a delicious twist to your carnivore meal plan.

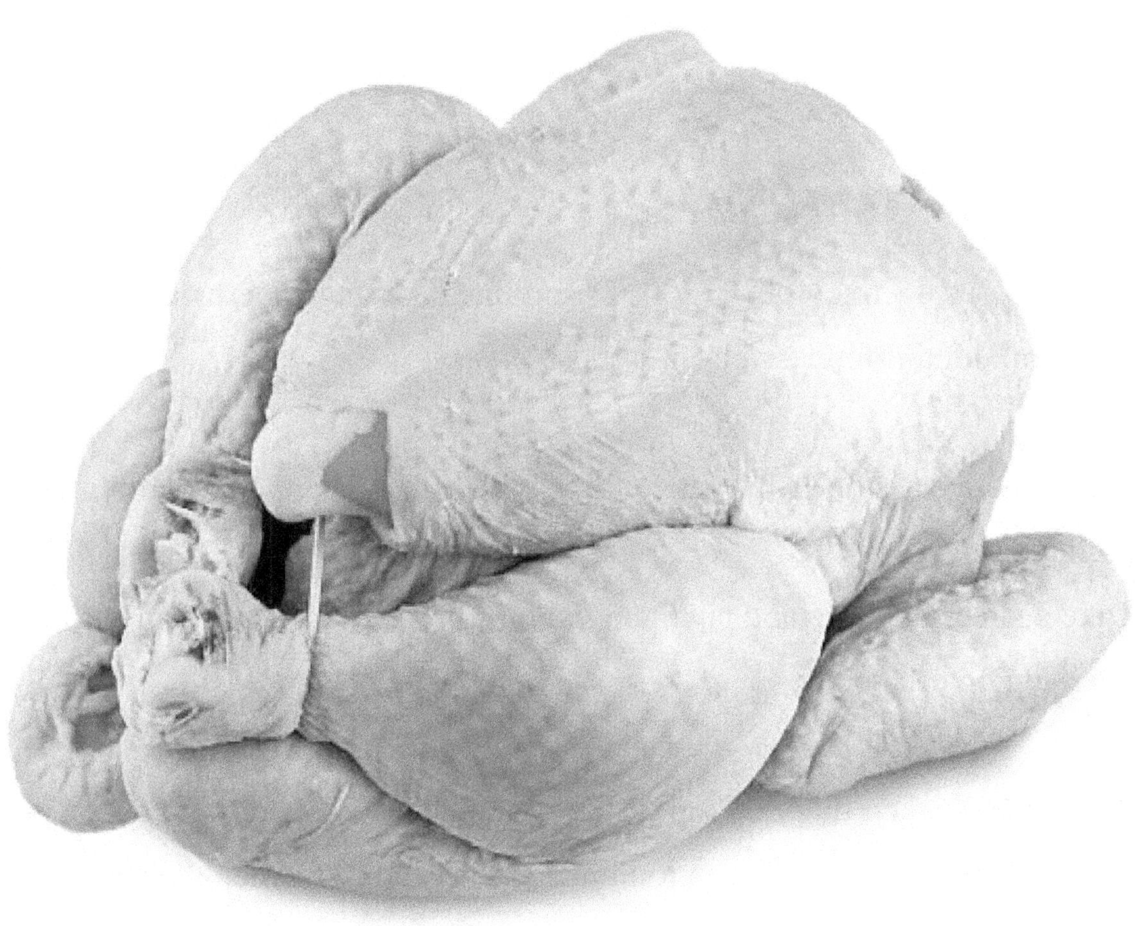

Bacon-Wrapped Chicken Thighs

Indulge in the irresistible combination of juicy chicken thighs wrapped in crispy bacon. This simple yet flavourful dish is perfect for a quick and satisfying carnivore meal.

Ingredients:

- 4 boneless, skinless chicken thighs
- slices of bacon
- Salt and pepper to taste

Step by Step Instructions:

1. Preheat your oven to 400°F (200°C) and line a baking sheet with parchment paper or aluminum foil for easy cleanup.

2. Season both sides of each chicken thigh with salt and pepper according to your taste preferences.

3. Take 2 slices of bacon and lay them flat on a cutting board or clean surface, slightly overlapping each other.

4. Place one chicken thigh on top of the bacon slices and wrap the bacon around the chicken thigh, securing it with toothpicks if necessary to keep the bacon in place.

5. Repeat this process for the remaining chicken thighs and bacon slices.

6   Arrange the bacon-wrapped chicken thighs on the prepared baking sheet, making sure they are evenly spaced apart.

7   Bake in the preheated oven for 25-30 minutes, or until the bacon is crispy and the chicken thighs are cooked through with an internal temperature of 165°F (75°C).

8   Once cooked, remove the bacon-wrapped chicken thighs from the oven and let them rest for a few minutes before serving.

9   Serve the bacon-wrapped chicken thighs hot and enjoy the delicious combination of juicy chicken and crispy bacon!

This simple yet delicious recipe for Bacon-Wrapped Chicken Thighs is sure to become a favorite in your carnivore meal rotation. Enjoy the irresistible flavors and satisfying textures of this carnivore delight!

Turkey Meatballs in Marinara Sauce

Treat yourself to these flavourful turkey meatballs simmered in rich marinara sauce. Packed with protein and bursting with Italian flavours, these meatballs are a carnivore-friendly twist on a classic favourite.

Ingredients:

For the Turkey Meatballs:

- 1-pound ground turkey

- 1/4 cup grated Parmesan cheese

- 1/4 cup almond flour (or any other low-carb flour substitute)

- 1 large egg

- 2 cloves garlic, minced

- 1 teaspoon dried oregano

- 1 teaspoon dried basil

- Salt and pepper to taste

For the Marinara Sauce:

- 2 tablespoons olive oil

- 1 onion, finely chopped

- 2 cloves garlic, minced

- 1 can (28 ounces) crushed tomatoes

- 1 teaspoon dried oregano

- 1 teaspoon dried basil

- Salt and pepper to taste

Step by Step Instructions:

1   In a large mixing bowl, combine the ground turkey, grated Parmesan cheese, almond flour, egg, minced garlic, dried oregano, dried basil, salt, and pepper. Mix until well combined.

2   Using your hands, shape the turkey mixture into meatballs of your desired size. Place the meatballs on a plate or baking sheet lined with parchment paper.

3   Heat olive oil in a large skillet over medium heat. Add the chopped onion and minced garlic, and sauté until softened and fragrant, about 3-4 minutes.

4   Stir in the crushed tomatoes, dried oregano, dried basil, salt, and pepper. Bring the sauce to a simmer and let it cook for about 10-15 minutes, allowing the flavors to meld together.

5   Carefully add the turkey meatballs to the simmering marinara sauce, making sure they are evenly distributed in the skillet.

6   Cover the skillet with a lid and let the meatballs simmer in the sauce for 15-20 minutes, or until cooked through with an internal temperature of 165°F (75°C).

7   Once the meatballs are cooked, remove the skillet from the heat and let it sit for a few minutes to allow the sauce to thicken slightly.

8   Serve the turkey meatballs hot with a generous spoonful of marinara sauce on top. Garnish with freshly chopped basil or parsley if desired.

9   Enjoy these flavorful turkey meatballs in marinara sauce as a delicious and satisfying carnivore-friendly meal!

This recipe for Turkey Meatballs in Marinara Sauce offers a delightful twist on a classic favorite, perfect for indulging in rich Italian flavors while sticking to your carnivore diet. Bon appétit!

Chicken Drumsticks with Paprika Seasoning

Enjoy the smoky and slightly spicy flavours of paprika-seasoned chicken drumsticks. These tender and flavourful drumsticks are perfect for a carnivore-friendly dinner that's both satisfying and delicious.

Ingredients:

- 6 chicken drumsticks
- 2 tablespoons olive oil
- 2 teaspoons smoked paprika
- 1 teaspoon garlic powder
- 1 teaspoon onion powder
- 1/2 teaspoon dried thyme
- 1/2 teaspoon dried oregano
- Salt and pepper to taste

Step by Step Instructions:

1   Preheat your oven to 400°F (200°C) and line a baking sheet with parchment paper or aluminum foil for easy cleanup.

2   In a small bowl, combine the smoked paprika, garlic powder, onion powder, dried thyme, dried oregano, salt, and pepper. Mix well to create the paprika seasoning.

3   Pat the chicken drumsticks dry with paper towels to remove any excess moisture. This will help the seasoning adhere better to the drumsticks.

4   Drizzle the olive oil over the chicken drumsticks and rub them evenly to coat them with the oil.

5   Sprinkle the paprika seasoning mixture over the chicken drumsticks, making sure to coat them evenly on all sides.

6   Place the seasoned chicken drumsticks on the prepared baking sheet, spacing them apart to allow for even cooking.

7   Bake the chicken drumsticks in the preheated oven for 35-40 minutes, or until they are golden brown and cooked through with an internal temperature of 165°F (75°C).

8   Once cooked, remove the chicken drumsticks from the oven and let them rest for a few minutes before serving.

9   Serve the chicken drumsticks hot and enjoy the smoky and slightly spicy flavors of this delicious carnivore-friendly dish!

These Chicken Drumsticks with Paprika Seasoning are sure to be a hit at your dinner table, offering tender and flavorful meat with a hint of smokiness and spice. Enjoy this simple yet satisfying carnivore meal!

Chicken Liver Sautéed in Butter

Experience the rich and buttery goodness of sautéed chicken liver. Packed with essential nutrients and delicious flavours, this simple dish is a carnivore delight that's both nutritious and satisfying.

Ingredients:

- 1-pound chicken livers, cleaned and trimmed
- 4 tablespoons unsalted butter
- 2 cloves garlic, minced
- Salt and pepper to taste
- Fresh parsley for garnish (optional)

Step by Step Instructions:

1   Rinse the chicken livers under cold water and pat them dry with paper towels.

Trim off any excess fat or connective tissue and cut the livers into bite-sized pieces if desired.

2   Heat 2 tablespoons of unsalted butter in a large skillet over medium heat until melted and sizzling.

3   Add the minced garlic to the skillet and sauté for 1-2 minutes, or until fragrant.

4   Carefully add the chicken livers to the skillet in a single layer, making sure not to overcrowd the pan. Cook the livers for 3-4 minutes on each side, or until browned and cooked through. Avoid overcooking to prevent the livers from becoming tough and rubbery.

5   Season the chicken livers generously with salt and pepper to taste while they are cooking in the skillet.

6   Once the chicken livers are cooked to your desired doneness, remove them from the skillet and transfer them to a serving plate or platter.

7   In the same skillet, add the remaining 2 tablespoons of unsalted butter and melt it over medium heat.

8   Pour the melted butter over the cooked chicken livers on the serving plate.

9 Garnish the sautéed chicken livers with fresh parsley for added flavor and presentation, if desired.

10 Serve the chicken livers hot and enjoy the rich and buttery goodness of this simple yet delicious carnivore delight!

This recipe for Chicken Liver Sautéed in Butter offers a decadent and nutrient-packed dish that's perfect for a satisfying carnivore meal. Enjoy the delicious flavors and nourishing benefits of this classic favorite!

Turkey Breast Roast with Herbs

Impress your taste buds with the succulent flavours of herb-roasted turkey breast. This tender and juicy roast is seasoned with aromatic herbs for a carnivore-friendly dish that's perfect for any occasion.

Ingredients:

- 1 boneless turkey breast (about 3-4 pounds)
- 4 tablespoons unsalted butter, melted
- 2 cloves garlic, minced
- 2 teaspoons dried thyme
- 2 teaspoons dried rosemary
- 2 teaspoons dried sage

- Salt and pepper to taste

- Fresh parsley for garnish (optional)

Step by Step Instructions:

1 Preheat your oven to 375°F (190°C) and grease a roasting pan or baking dish with non-stick cooking spray.

2 In a small bowl, combine the melted unsalted butter, minced garlic, dried thyme, dried rosemary, dried sage, salt, and pepper. Mix well to create the herb butter mixture.

3 Place the boneless turkey breast in the greased roasting pan or baking dish, skin side up.

4 Use your hands or a basting brush to coat the entire surface of the turkey breast with the herb butter mixture, ensuring it is evenly distributed.

5 Season the turkey breast generously with additional salt and pepper to taste.

6 Place the roasting pan or baking dish in the preheated oven and roast the turkey breast for approximately 1 1/2 to 2 hours, or until the internal temperature reaches 165°F (75°C) when measured with a meat thermometer.

7 Baste the turkey breast with the pan juices and herb butter mixture every 30 minutes during the cooking process to keep it moist and flavorful.

8   Once the turkey breast is fully cooked and golden brown on the outside, remove it from the oven and transfer it to a cutting board.

9   Allow the turkey breast to rest for 10-15 minutes before slicing to allow the juices to redistribute and the meat to become more tender.

10 Slice the herb-roasted turkey breast into thin slices and arrange them on a serving platter.

11 Garnish the sliced turkey breast with fresh parsley for added flavor and presentation, if desired.

12 Serve the herb-roasted turkey breast hot and enjoy the succulent flavors of this delicious carnivore-friendly dish!

This recipe for Turkey Breast Roast with Herbs offers a delightful twist on a classic favorite, perfect for impressing your taste buds with tender and juicy herb-roasted turkey breast. Enjoy the aromatic flavors and succulent textures of this irresistible carnivore delight!

Turkey Bacon-Wrapped Jalapeño Poppers

Kick up the heat with these spicy turkey bacon-wrapped jalapeño poppers.

Stuffed with creamy cheese and wrapped in crispy bacon, these poppers are a carnivore-friendly appetizer that's bursting with flavour.

Ingredients:

- large jalapeño peppers, halved lengthwise and seeds removed
- slices turkey bacon, cut in half crosswise
- 4 ounces' cream cheese, softened
- 1/2 cup shredded cheddar cheese
- 1/2 teaspoon garlic powder
- 1/2 teaspoon onion powder
- Salt and pepper to taste
- Toothpicks (optional, for securing the bacon)

Step by Step Instructions:

1 Preheat your oven to 400°F (200°C) and line a baking sheet with parchment paper or aluminum foil for easy cleanup.

2 In a small bowl, mix together the softened cream cheese, shredded cheddar cheese, garlic powder, onion powder, salt, and pepper until well combined. This will be the filling for the jalapeño poppers.

3 Fill each jalapeño pepper half with a generous amount of the cream cheese mixture, ensuring they are evenly filled.

4 Wrap each cream cheese-filled jalapeño half with a half-slice of turkey bacon, ensuring the bacon is tightly wrapped around the pepper. You can secure the bacon with toothpicks if needed.

5 Place the bacon-wrapped jalapeño poppers on the prepared baking sheet, seam side down, and arrange them in a single layer.

6 Bake the jalapeño poppers in the preheated oven for 20-25 minutes, or until the bacon is crispy and golden brown.

7 Once cooked, remove the jalapeño poppers from the oven and let them cool slightly before serving.

8 Serve the turkey bacon-wrapped jalapeño poppers hot as a delicious and flavorful appetizer or snack.

These Turkey Bacon-Wrapped Jalapeño Poppers are sure to be a hit at your next gathering, offering a perfect combination of spicy jalapeños, creamy cheese filling, and crispy bacon. Enjoy these carnivore-friendly poppers as a delicious and satisfying appetizer!

Turkey Sausage Patties with Sage

Start your day off right with these flavourful turkey sausage patties seasoned with aromatic sage. These homemade patties are a delicious and protein-packed addition to your carnivore breakfast.

Ingredients:

- 1-pound ground turkey
- 2 tablespoons fresh sage, finely chopped
- 1 teaspoon garlic powder
- 1 teaspoon onion powder
- 1/2 teaspoon paprika
- 1/2 teaspoon salt
- 1/4 teaspoon black pepper
- 1 tablespoon olive oil (for cooking)

Step by Step Instructions

1 In a large mixing bowl, combine the ground turkey, finely chopped fresh sage, garlic powder, onion powder, paprika, salt, and black pepper. Mix well until all the ingredients are evenly incorporated.

2 Divide the seasoned turkey mixture into equal portions and shape them into round patties, about 2-3 inches in diameter and 1/2 inch thick. You should be able to make approximately 8-10 patties, depending on the size.

3 Heat the olive oil in a large skillet or frying pan over medium heat.

4 Once the skillet is hot, carefully add the turkey sausage patties in a single layer, making sure not to overcrowd the pan.

You may need to cook the patties in batches, depending on the size of your skillet.

5 Cook the turkey sausage patties for 3-4 minutes on each side, or until they are golden brown and cooked through. Use a spatula to flip the patties halfway through the cooking process to ensure even browning.

6 Once the turkey sausage patties are fully cooked and browned on both sides, transfer them to a plate lined with paper towels to drain any excess grease.

7 Repeat the cooking process with the remaining turkey sausage patties until all the patties are cooked.

8 Serve the turkey sausage patties hot as a delicious and protein-packed addition to your carnivore breakfast or any meal of the day.

These Turkey Sausage Patties with Sage are bursting with flavorful herbs and spices, making them a perfect savory option for starting your day off right. Enjoy these homemade patties as a satisfying and nutritious addition to your carnivore meal plan!

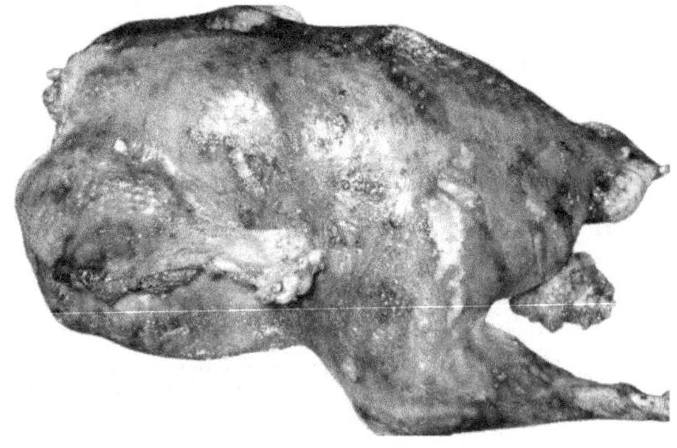

Chapter 5

PORK PARADISE

Pork lovers rejoice! In this chapter, we explore the mouthwatering world of pork dishes that will tantalize your taste buds and keep you satisfied on your carnivore journey. From succulent tenderloins to crispy belly slices, pork offers a variety of cuts that can be prepared in deliciously different ways. Let's dive into the pork paradise and discover a range of flavorful recipes that celebrate this versatile meat.

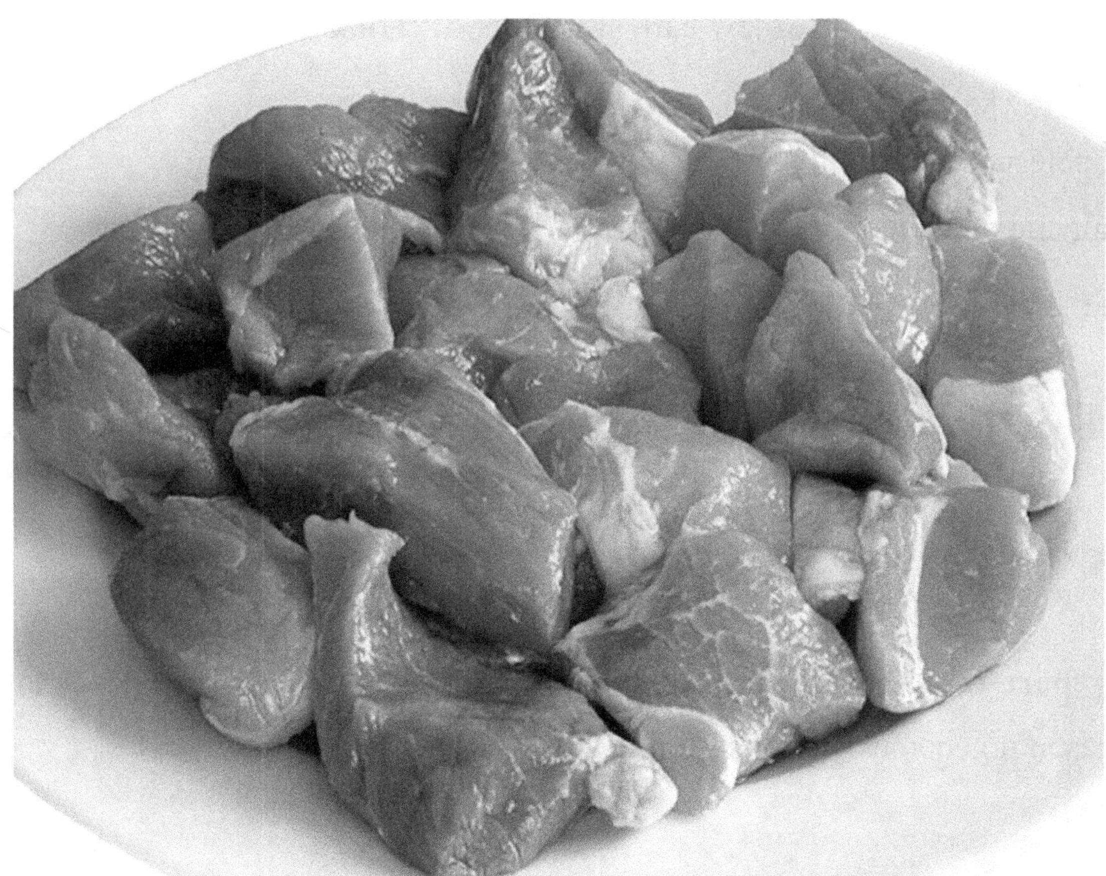

Pork Tenderloin with Mustard Glaze

Delight in the tender goodness of pork tenderloin coated with a tangy mustard glaze, creating a perfect harmony of flavors in every bite.

Ingredients:

- 1 pork tenderloin (about 1 to 1.5 pounds)
- 2 tablespoons Dijon mustard
- 2 tablespoons whole grain mustard
- 2 tablespoons honey (or low-carb sweetener of choice)
- 2 cloves garlic, minced
- 1 tablespoon olive oil
- Salt and pepper to taste
- Fresh parsley for garnish (optional)

Step by Step Instructions:

1 **Preheat the oven:** Preheat your oven to 400°F (200°C).

2 **Prepare the pork tenderloin:** Pat the pork tenderloin dry with paper towels and season it generously with salt and pepper on all sides.

3 **Make the mustard glaze:** In a small bowl, whisk together the Dijon mustard, whole grain mustard, honey, minced garlic, and olive oil until well combined.

4 **Coat the pork tenderloin:** Place the seasoned pork tenderloin in a roasting pan or baking dish. Spoon the mustard glaze over the pork tenderloin, spreading it evenly to coat the entire surface.

5 **Roast the pork tenderloin:** Roast the pork tenderloin in the preheated oven for about 20-25 minutes, or until the internal temperature reaches 145°F (63°C) for medium-rare or 160°F (71°C) for medium. Baste the pork with the glaze halfway through cooking.

6 **Rest and slice:** Once cooked to your desired doneness, remove the pork tenderloin from the oven and let it rest for 5-10 minutes before slicing. This allows the juices to redistribute, resulting in a juicy and tender pork.

7 **Slice and serve:** Slice the pork tenderloin into thick slices and arrange them on a serving platter. Garnish with fresh parsley if desired. Serve warm and enjoy the tender goodness of pork tenderloin with tangy mustard glaze!

This Pork Tenderloin with Mustard Glaze is a perfect dish for any occasion, whether it's a weeknight dinner or a special gathering. With its flavorful glaze and tender meat, it's sure to become a favorite in your carnivore recipe collection.

Pork Belly Slices with Crispy Skin

Indulge in the crispy, golden-brown skin and melt-in-your-mouth meat of pork belly slices, a carnivore's dream come true.

Ingredients:

- 1 lb. pork belly, skin-on
- Salt, to taste
- Pepper, to taste

Step by step Instructions:

1 **Preheat the oven:** Preheat your oven to 425°F (220°C).

2 **Prepare the pork belly:** Pat the pork belly dry with paper towels. Using a sharp knife, score the skin of the pork belly in a crosshatch pattern, being careful not to cut through the meat.

3 **Season the pork belly:** Season the pork belly generously with salt and pepper on both sides, including the skin.

4 **Roast the pork belly:** Place the pork belly on a wire rack set over a baking sheet, with the skin side facing up. This allows the heat to circulate evenly around the pork belly, ensuring crispy skin. Roast in the preheated oven for about 30-40 minutes, or until the skin is crispy and golden brown, and the meat is tender and cooked through.

5   **Broil for extra crispiness (optional):** If desired, after roasting, you can switch the oven to broil and broil the pork belly for an additional 2-3 minutes to further crisp up the skin. Keep a close eye on it to prevent burning.

6   **Rest and slice:** Once cooked to perfection, remove the pork belly from the oven and let it rest for a few minutes before slicing. This allows the juices to redistribute, resulting in a juicy and flavorful pork belly.

7   **Slice and serve:** Slice the pork belly into thick slices, and serve hot as a delicious carnivore-friendly meal. Enjoy the crispy, golden-brown skin and melt-in-your-mouth meat of these pork belly slices - a true indulgence for any carnivore enthusiast!

Pork Shoulder Slow-Cooked in Its Own Juices

Experience the rich and savory taste of pork shoulder as it slow-cooks to perfection in its own juices, resulting in tender and flavorful meat that falls off the bone.

Ingredients:

- 3-4 lbs. pork shoulder (also known as pork butt), bone-in or boneless
- Salt, to taste
- Pepper, to taste

Step by Step Instructions:

1 **Preheat the oven:** Preheat your oven to 300°F (150°C).

2 **Prepare the pork shoulder:** Pat the pork shoulder dry with paper towels and season generously with salt and pepper on all sides.

3 **Place in roasting pan:** Place the seasoned pork shoulder in a roasting pan or oven-safe dish large enough to accommodate it.

4 **Cover tightly:** Cover the roasting pan tightly with aluminum foil, ensuring a snug fit to trap the juices inside.

5 **Slow cook:** Transfer the covered roasting pan to the preheated oven and slow-cook the pork shoulder for approximately 4-5 hours, or until the meat is fork-tender and easily falls apart.

6 **Check for doneness:** After the initial cooking time, carefully remove the foil and check the pork shoulder for doneness. The meat should be tender and easily shred with a fork.

7 **Baste with juices (optional):** If desired, baste the pork shoulder with its own juices periodically throughout the cooking process to keep it moist and flavorful.

8 **Rest and shred:** Once cooked to perfection, remove the pork shoulder from the oven and let it rest for a few minutes. Then, using two forks or meat claws, shred the pork shoulder into bite-sized pieces, discarding any excess fat or bone.

9   **Serve and enjoy:** Serve the tender and flavorful shredded pork shoulder hot as a hearty carnivore meal, or use it as a versatile ingredient in various dishes such as tacos, sandwiches, or salads. Enjoy the rich and savory taste of pork shoulder slow-cooked to perfection in its own juices!

Pork Loin Chops with Apple Cider Vinegar Glaze

Elevate pork loin chops with a sweet and tangy apple cider vinegar glaze, adding a burst of flavor to this classic cut of meat.

Ingredients:

- 4 pork loin chops, about 1-inch thick
- Salt, to taste
- Black pepper, to taste
- 1 tablespoon olive oil
- 1/4 cup apple cider vinegar
- 2 tablespoons honey (or sugar-free alternative for strict carnivore)
- 2 cloves garlic, minced
- 1 teaspoon dried thyme (optional)

Step by Step Instructions:

1 **Season the pork chops:** Season both sides of the pork loin chops with salt and black pepper according to your taste preferences.

2 **Heat the olive oil:** In a large skillet, heat the olive oil over medium-high heat until hot but not smoking.

3 **Sear the pork chops:** Carefully add the seasoned pork loin chops to the skillet and sear them for about 3-4 minutes on each side, or until they develop a golden-brown crust. Adjust the heat as needed to prevent burning.

4 **Make the glaze:** While the pork chops are searing, prepare the glaze. In a small bowl, combine the apple cider vinegar, honey, minced garlic, and dried thyme (if using). Mix well to combine.

5 **Add the glaze:** Once the pork chops are seared on both sides, pour the apple cider vinegar glaze over them in the skillet.

6 **Simmer:** Reduce the heat to medium-low and allow the pork chops to simmer in the glaze for an additional 5-7 minutes, or until they are cooked through and reach an internal temperature of 145°F (63°C) for medium doneness.

7 **Baste the chops:** Occasionally spoon the glaze from the skillet over the pork chops as they cook to ensure they are evenly coated and infused with flavor.

8   **Serve:** Once the pork chops are cooked to your desired level of doneness and the glaze has thickened slightly, remove them from the skillet and transfer them to a serving platter.

9   **Garnish and enjoy:** Garnish the pork chops with any remaining glaze from the skillet, and serve them hot with your favorite side dishes. Enjoy the sweet and tangy flavor of pork loin chops with apple cider vinegar glaze!

Pork Ribs Slow-Cooked with Dry Rub Seasoning

Dive into a rack of succulent pork ribs coated in a mouthwatering dry rub seasoning, offering a perfect balance of smoky, savory, and slightly sweet flavors.

Ingredients:

- 2 racks of pork ribs (baby back or spare ribs)
- 1/4 cup brown sugar (or sugar-free alternative for strict carnivore)
- 2 tablespoons paprika
- 1 tablespoon garlic powder
- 1 tablespoon onion powder
- 1 tablespoon chili powder
- 1 tablespoon salt
- 1 teaspoon black pepper
- 1/2 teaspoon cayenne pepper (optional, for added heat)

- 1/4 cup apple cider vinegar (for basting, optional)

Step by Step Instructions:

1 **Prepare the dry rub:** In a small bowl, combine the brown sugar, paprika, garlic powder, onion powder, chili powder, salt, black pepper, and cayenne pepper (if using). Mix well to ensure all the spices are evenly incorporated.

2 **Prepare the ribs:** Remove the membrane from the back of the ribs if desired, then pat the ribs dry with paper towels. This will help the dry rub adhere better to the meat.

3 **Apply the dry rub:** Generously sprinkle the dry rub mixture over both sides of the ribs, rubbing it into the meat to ensure even coverage. Use your hands to press the seasoning into the meat for better flavor penetration.

4 **Preheat the oven:** Preheat your oven to 275°F (135°C) to slow-cook the ribs.

5 **Wrap and refrigerate:** Wrap the seasoned ribs tightly in aluminum foil or plastic wrap and refrigerate them for at least 1 hour, or overnight if possible. This allows the flavors to meld and marinate the meat.

6 **Slow-cook the ribs:** Place the wrapped ribs on a baking sheet and transfer them to the preheated oven. Slow-cook the ribs for 2.5 to 3 hours, or until the meat is tender and easily pulls away from the bones.

7. **Optional basting:** If desired, you can baste the ribs with apple cider vinegar every hour during the cooking process to add moisture and enhance flavor.

8. **Finish on the grill (optional):** For added flavor and texture, you can finish the ribs on the grill over medium-high heat for 10-15 minutes, basting with any remaining juices or sauce.

9. **Rest and serve:** Once the ribs are cooked to perfection, remove them from the oven (or grill) and let them rest for a few minutes before slicing between the bones. Serve hot and enjoy the irresistible flavor of slow-cooked pork ribs with dry rub seasoning!

Pork Belly Burnt Ends

Indulge in the irresistible combination of caramelized pork belly burnt ends, offering a delightful contrast of crispy exterior and tender, juicy interior.

Ingredients:

- 2 lbs. pork belly, skin removed
- 1/4 cup brown sugar (or sugar-free alternative for strict carnivore)
- 2 tablespoons paprika
- 1 tablespoon garlic powder
- 1 tablespoon onion powder
- 1 tablespoon salt

- 1 teaspoon black pepper

- 1/2 teaspoon cayenne pepper (optional, for added heat)

- 1/4 cup apple cider vinegar

- 1/4 cup water

- 1/2 cup carnivore-friendly barbecue sauce (optional)

Step by Step Instructions:

1 **Preheat the smoker:** Preheat your smoker to 250°F (120°C). If you don't have a smoker, you can use an oven with a wire rack set over a baking sheet.

2 **Prepare the pork belly:** Cut the pork belly into bite-sized cubes, approximately 1 to 1.5 inches in size.

3 **Create the dry rub:** In a bowl, mix together the brown sugar, paprika, garlic powder, onion powder, salt, black pepper, and cayenne pepper (if using).

4 **Coat the pork belly:** Sprinkle the dry rub generously over the pork belly cubes, ensuring each piece is well-coated. Use your hands to massage the rub into the meat.

5 **Smoke the pork belly:** Place the seasoned pork belly cubes directly on the smoker grates or on the wire rack in the oven. Smoke them at 250°F for 2.5 to 3 hours, or until they develop a caramelized crust.

6 **Make the braising liquid:** In a bowl, mix together the apple cider vinegar and water to create a braising liquid.

7 **Braise the burnt ends:** Transfer the smoked pork belly cubes to a disposable aluminum pan and pour the braising liquid over them. Cover the pan tightly with foil.

8 **Continue cooking:** Return the pan to the smoker or oven and continue cooking for an additional 1.5 to 2 hours, or until the burnt ends are tender and flavorful.

9 **Optional sauce:** If desired, you can brush the burnt ends with a carnivore-friendly barbecue sauce during the last 30 minutes of cooking for added flavor.

10 **Serve and enjoy:** Once the pork belly burnt ends are done, remove them from the smoker or oven. Allow them to rest for a few minutes before serving. The result is a delightful dish with crispy exteriors and juicy interiors—perfect for indulging in pork paradise!

Pork Cracklings

Crispy, crunchy, and utterly addictive, pork cracklings are the ultimate carnivore snack, providing a satisfying crunch with every bite.

Ingredients:

- 1 lb. pork skin, cleaned and dried

- Salt, to taste

Step by Step Instructions:

1 **Prepare the pork skin:** Ensure the pork skin is thoroughly cleaned and dried. You can ask your butcher to provide you with pork skin specifically for cracklings or use leftover pork skin from other cuts of meat.

2 **Preheat the oven:** Preheat your oven to 375°F (190°C) and line a baking sheet with parchment paper or aluminum foil for easy cleanup.

3 **Score the pork skin:** Using a sharp knife or razor blade, score the pork skin into small squares or rectangles. Be careful not to cut all the way through the skin, as you want to create shallow cuts to facilitate the rendering process.

4 **Season with salt:** Sprinkle the scored pork skin generously with salt, ensuring that each piece is evenly coated. The salt will help draw out moisture from the skin and aid in the crisping process.

5 **Bake in the oven:** Place the seasoned pork skin pieces on the prepared baking sheet, making sure they are in a single layer and not overlapping. Bake in the preheated oven for 30-40 minutes, or until the pork skin is golden brown and crispy.

6 **Check for doneness:** Keep a close eye on the pork cracklings as they bake, as they can quickly go from crispy to burnt.

You'll know they're done when they are uniformly golden brown and crispy all over.

7   **Remove from the oven:** Once the pork cracklings are done, remove them from the oven and let them cool slightly on the baking sheet. They will continue to crisp up as they cool.

8   **Serve and enjoy:** Serve the pork cracklings warm as a delicious and crunchy carnivore snack. Enjoy their irresistible crispiness and savory flavor with every bite!

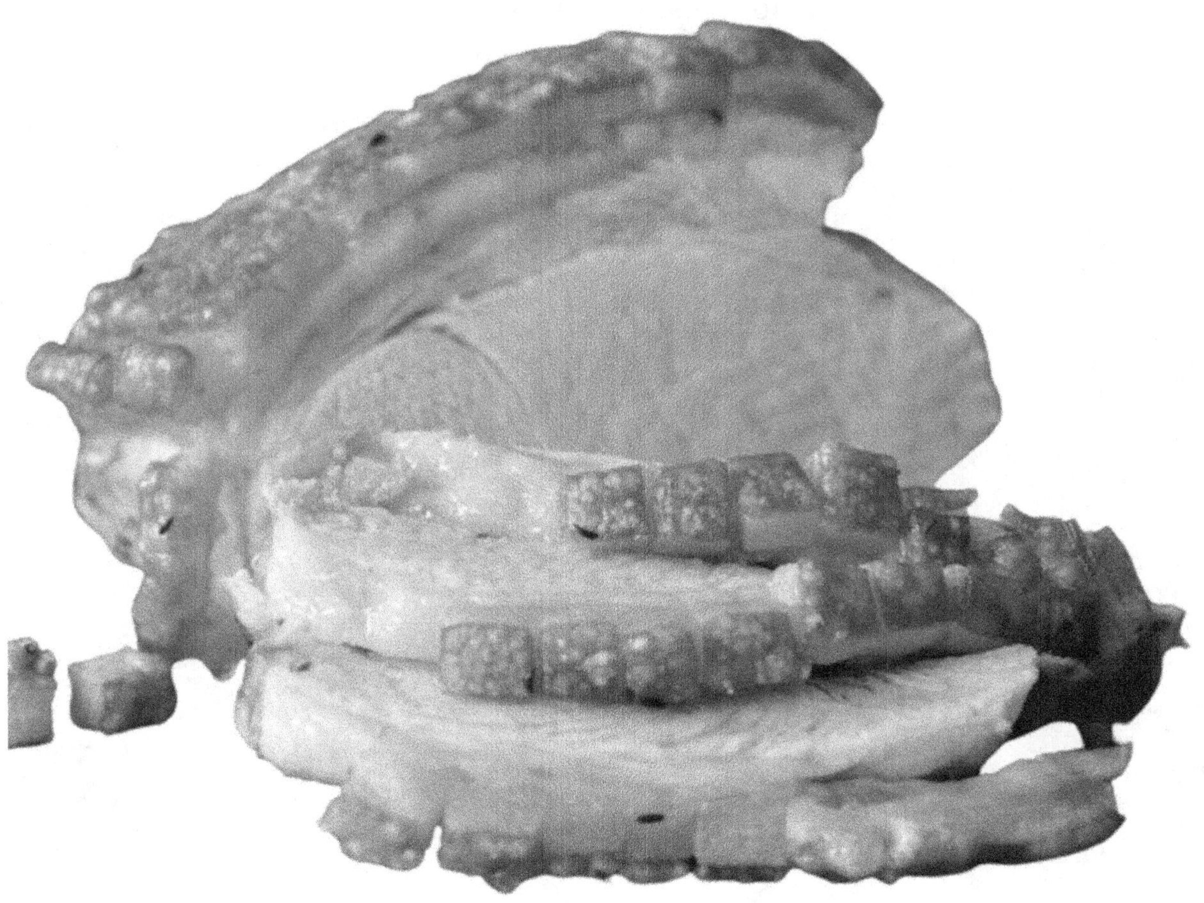

LAMB LOVE

Lamb, with its distinctive flavor and tender texture, offers a delightful array of dishes for carnivores to enjoy. From succulent chops to hearty shanks, lamb dishes are sure to tantalize your taste buds and provide a satisfying meal experience. In this chapter, we explore a variety of mouthwatering lamb recipes that showcase the versatility and deliciousness of this beloved meat.

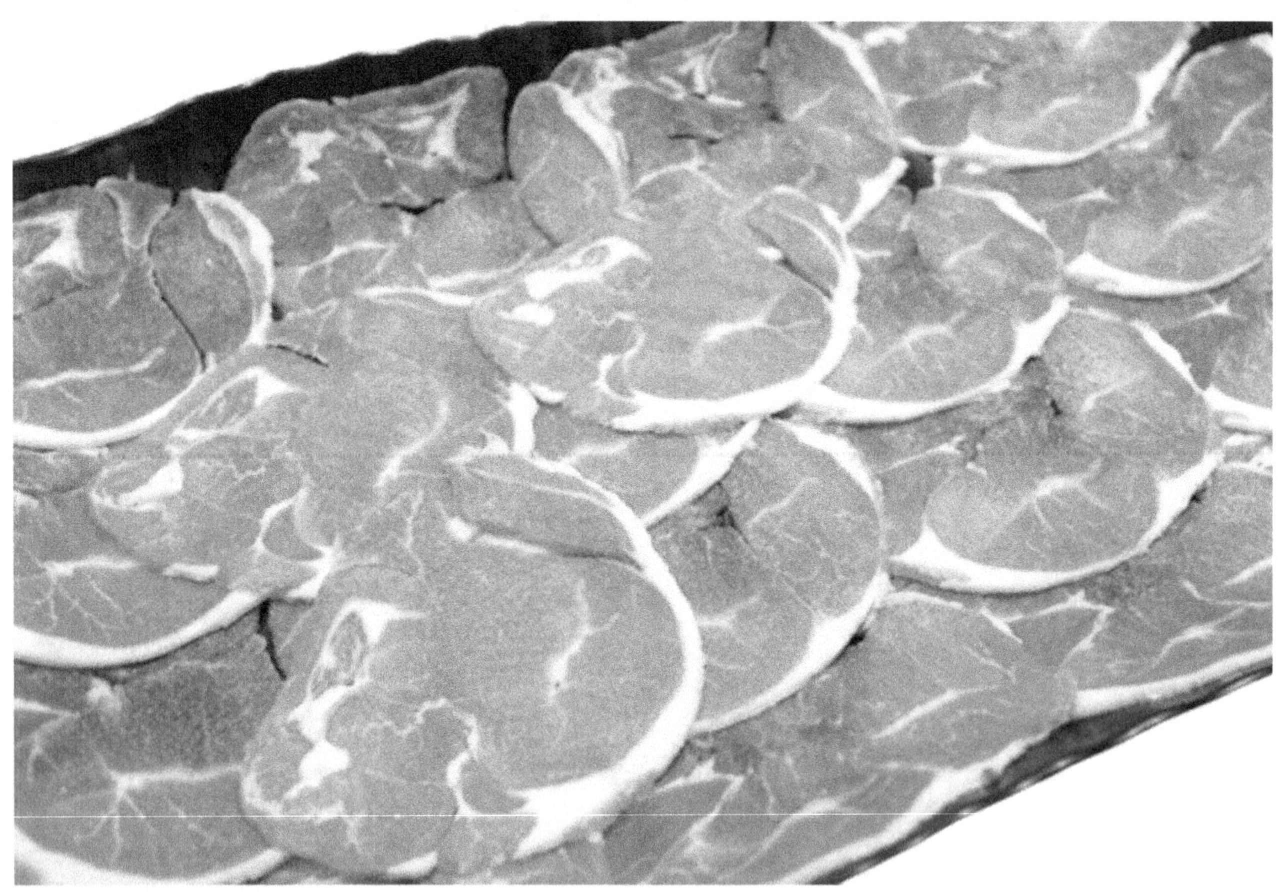

Lamb Chops with Rosemary

Full of flavor and tenderness, lamb chops seasoned with aromatic rosemary are a classic carnivore delight. Serve them alongside your favorite low-carb vegetables for a complete and satisfying meal.

Ingredients:

- 4 lamb chops
- 2 tablespoons olive oil
- 2 cloves garlic, minced
- 2 tablespoons fresh rosemary, chopped
- Salt and pepper to taste

Step by Step Instructions:

1 **Preheat the Oven:** Preheat your oven to 400°F (200°C).

2 **Prepare the Lamb Chops:** Pat dry the lamb chops with paper towels to remove excess moisture. This helps ensure a crispy exterior when cooking.

3 **Season the Lamb Chops:** In a small bowl, combine the olive oil, minced garlic, chopped rosemary, salt, and pepper. Rub this mixture evenly over both sides of the lamb chops, ensuring they are well coated with the seasoning.

4 **Sear the Lamb Chops:** Heat a skillet over medium-high heat. Once hot, add the lamb chops to the skillet and sear for 2-3 minutes on each side, or until they develop a golden-brown crust.

5 **Transfer to the Oven:** Transfer the seared lamb chops to a baking dish or oven-safe skillet and place them in the preheated oven.

6 **Roast the Lamb Chops:** Roast the lamb chops in the oven for 10-12 minutes for medium-rare, or longer if desired, depending on your preferred level of doneness.

7 **Rest and Serve:** Once cooked to your liking, remove the lamb chops from the oven and let them rest for a few minutes before serving. This allows the juices to redistribute and ensures tender, juicy meat.

8 **Serve:** Serve the lamb chops alongside your favorite low-carb vegetables or salad for a complete and satisfying carnivore meal. Enjoy the flavorful and tender lamb chops seasoned with aromatic rosemary.

Braised Lamb Shank in Red Wine

Tender and falling-off-the-bone, braised lamb shank cooked in red wine is a comforting and elegant dish perfect for special occasions or a cozy night in. The rich flavors of the wine complement the savory lamb, creating a truly indulgent experience.

Ingredients:

- 4 lamb shanks

- 2 tablespoons olive oil

- 1 onion, diced

- 2 carrots, diced

- 2 celery stalks, diced

- 4 cloves garlic, minced

- 2 cups red wine (such as Cabernet Sauvignon or Merlot)

- 2 cups beef or chicken broth

- 2 tablespoons tomato paste

- 2 sprigs fresh rosemary

- Salt and pepper to taste

Step by Step Instructions:

1 **Preheat the Oven:** Preheat your oven to 325°F (160°C).

2 **Brown the Lamb Shanks:** Heat olive oil in a large oven-safe Dutch oven or heavy-bottomed pot over medium-high heat. Season the lamb shanks with salt and pepper, then brown them on all sides in the hot oil. This will take about 8-10 minutes. Once browned, remove the lamb shanks from the pot and set them aside.

3 **Sauté the Vegetables:** In the same pot, add diced onion, carrots, and celery. Sauté until softened, about 5-7 minutes. Add minced garlic and sauté for an additional 1-2 minutes until fragrant.

4   **Deglaze the Pot:** Pour in the red wine and scrape the bottom of the pot to deglaze, loosening any browned bits stuck to the bottom. Allow the wine to simmer for a few minutes to reduce slightly.

5   **Add Remaining Ingredients:** Stir in the beef or chicken broth, tomato paste, and fresh rosemary sprigs. Return the browned lamb shanks to the pot, nestling them into the liquid and vegetables.

6   **Braise the Lamb Shanks:** Cover the pot with a lid and transfer it to the preheated oven. Allow the lamb shanks to braise in the oven for 2.5 to 3 hours, or until the meat is tender and falling off the bone.

7   **Serve:** Once the lamb shanks are done braising, carefully remove them from the pot and transfer to a serving platter. Spoon the vegetables and sauce over the lamb shanks. Serve hot and enjoy the rich and flavorful braised lamb shanks cooked in red wine.

Lamb Kebabs with Mint Yogurt Sauce

These succulent lamb kebabs, marinated in fragrant spices and grilled to perfection, are paired with a refreshing mint yogurt sauce for a burst of flavor. Whether served as an appetizer or main course, these kebabs are sure to impress.

Ingredients:

For the Lamb Kebabs:

- 1 lb. (450g) lamb leg or shoulder, trimmed and cut into 1-inch cubes

- 2 tablespoons olive oil

- 2 cloves garlic, minced

- 1 teaspoon ground cumin

- 1 teaspoon ground coriander

- 1 teaspoon paprika

- 1/2 teaspoon ground turmeric

- Salt and pepper to taste

- Wooden or metal skewers

For the Mint Yogurt Sauce:

- 1 cup Greek yogurt

- 1/4 cup fresh mint leaves, finely chopped

- 1 tablespoon lemon juice

- 1 clove garlic, minced

- Salt and pepper to taste

Step by Step Instructions:

1 **Marinate the Lamb:** In a bowl, combine olive oil, minced garlic, ground cumin, ground coriander, paprika, ground turmeric, salt, and pepper.

Add the cubed lamb to the marinade, ensuring it's evenly coated. Cover and refrigerate for at least 1 hour, or ideally overnight, to allow the flavors to meld.

2 **Prepare the Skewers:** If using wooden skewers, soak them in water for about 30 minutes to prevent them from burning on the grill. Thread the marinated lamb cubes onto the skewers, leaving a small space between each piece.

3 **Preheat the Grill:** Preheat your grill to medium-high heat. Brush the grates with oil to prevent sticking.

4 **Grill the Kebabs:** Place the lamb kebabs on the preheated grill and cook for 8-10 minutes, turning occasionally, until the lamb is cooked to your desired doneness and has developed grill marks on all sides.

5 **Make the Mint Yogurt Sauce:** While the kebabs are grilling, prepare the mint yogurt sauce. In a small bowl, combine Greek yogurt, finely chopped mint leaves, lemon juice, minced garlic, salt, and pepper. Mix well until smooth and creamy.

6 **Serve:** Once the lamb kebabs are cooked, remove them from the grill and transfer to a serving platter.

7 Serve hot with the mint yogurt sauce on the side for dipping or drizzling. Enjoy the succulent lamb kebabs with a refreshing burst of flavor from the mint yogurt sauce.

Lamb Burgers with Tzatziki Sauce

Elevate your burger game with juicy lamb burgers topped with creamy tzatziki sauce. These flavorful burgers offer a Mediterranean twist on a classic favorite, perfect for a casual dinner or weekend barbecue.

Ingredients:

For the Lamb Burgers:

- 1 lb. (450g) ground lamb
- 1/4 cup finely chopped red onion
- 2 cloves garlic, minced
- 1 tablespoon fresh mint, finely chopped
- 1 tablespoon fresh parsley, finely chopped
- 1 teaspoon ground cumin
- 1 teaspoon ground coriander
- 1/2 teaspoon paprika
- Salt and pepper to taste
- Olive oil for grilling
- Burger buns or lettuce wraps (optional)

For the Tzatziki Sauce:

- 1 cup Greek yogurt
- 1/2 cucumber, grated and squeezed to remove excess moisture

- 1 clove garlic, minced

- 1 tablespoon fresh dill, chopped

- 1 tablespoon lemon juice

- Salt and pepper to taste

Step by Step Instructions:

1 **Prepare the Tzatziki Sauce:** In a small bowl, combine Greek yogurt, grated cucumber, minced garlic, chopped dill, lemon juice, salt, and pepper. Mix well until all ingredients are thoroughly combined. Cover and refrigerate the tzatziki sauce for at least 30 minutes to allow the flavors to meld.

2 **Make the Lamb Burgers:** In a large mixing bowl, combine ground lamb, finely chopped red onion, minced garlic, chopped mint, chopped parsley, ground cumin, ground coriander, paprika, salt, and pepper. Mix until all ingredients are evenly incorporated.

3 **Form the Burger Patties:** Divide the lamb mixture into 4 equal portions and shape each portion into a burger patty, about 1/2-inch thick. Make a slight indentation in the center of each patty to prevent it from bulging during cooking.

4 **Preheat the Grill:** Preheat your grill or grill pan to medium-high heat. Brush the grates with olive oil to prevent sticking.

5 **Grill the Lamb Burgers:** Place the burger patties on the preheated grill and cook for 4-5 minutes per side, or until they reach your desired level of doneness. Avoid pressing down on the patties while cooking to retain their juices.

6 **Assemble the Burgers:** If using burger buns, lightly toast them on the grill. Place a grilled lamb burger patty on each bun and top with a generous spoonful of tzatziki sauce. Alternatively, use lettuce wraps for a low-carb option.

7 **Serve:** Serve the lamb burgers with tzatziki sauce alongside your favorite side dishes, such as Greek salad or roasted vegetables. Enjoy the juicy and flavorful lamb burgers with the refreshing taste of homemade tzatziki sauce.

Lamb Liver Sautéed in Bacon Fat

Lamb liver, cooked in savory bacon fat, is a nutrient-dense dish that provides essential vitamins and minerals. Savor the rich flavors of this hearty organ meat for a satisfying and nourishing meal.

Ingredients:

- 1 lb. lamb liver, sliced
- 4 slices bacon
- Salt and pepper to taste
- Optional: fresh herbs for garnish

Step by Step Instructions:

1   **Prepare the Lamb Liver:** Rinse the lamb liver slices under cold water and pat them dry with paper towels. Season both sides of the liver slices with salt and pepper according to your taste preferences.

2   **Cook the Bacon:** In a large skillet or frying pan, cook the bacon slices over medium heat until they are crispy and golden brown. This will take about 5-7 minutes per side. Once cooked, remove the bacon from the pan and set it aside on a plate lined with paper towels to drain excess grease. Reserve the bacon fat in the skillet for cooking the lamb liver.

3   **Sauté the Lamb Liver:** Increase the heat to medium-high and carefully place the seasoned lamb liver slices in the skillet with the rendered bacon fat. Cook the liver slices for about 2-3 minutes on each side, or until they are browned and cooked through. Be cautious not to overcook the liver, as it can become tough and dry.

4   **Serve:** Once the lamb liver slices are cooked to your desired doneness, transfer them to a serving platter. Crumble the cooked bacon slices over the top of the liver slices for added flavor and texture. Garnish with fresh herbs if desired, and serve immediately while hot.

5   **Enjoy:** Savor the rich and savory flavors of the lamb liver sautéed in bacon fat as a nourishing and satisfying meal. Pair it with your favorite side dishes, such as roasted vegetables or a simple salad, for a complete carnivore-friendly feast.

Grilled Lamb Leg Steaks

Grilled lamb leg steaks, seasoned with herbs and spices, are a simple yet delicious way to enjoy the bold flavors of lamb. Serve them with a side salad or roasted vegetables for a wholesome and satisfying meal.

Ingredients:

- 4 lamb leg steaks, about 1 inch thick
- 2 tablespoons olive oil
- 2 cloves garlic, minced
- 1 tablespoon fresh rosemary, finely chopped
- 1 tablespoon fresh thyme, finely chopped
- 1 teaspoon paprika
- Salt and pepper to taste

Step by Step Instructions:

1 **Prepare the Marinade:** In a small bowl, combine the olive oil, minced garlic, chopped rosemary, chopped thyme, paprika, salt, and pepper. Mix well to combine.

2 **Marinate the Lamb Steaks:** Place the lamb leg steaks in a shallow dish or a resalable plastic bag.

Pour the marinade over the steaks, making sure they are evenly coated. Cover the dish or seal the bag, and refrigerate for at least 30 minutes to allow the flavors to meld.

3 **Preheat the Grill:** Preheat your grill to medium-high heat. If using a gas grill, preheat for about 10-15 minutes. If using a charcoal grill, light the charcoal and let it burn until the coals are covered with white ash.

4 **Grill the Lamb Steaks:** Remove the marinated lamb leg steaks from the refrigerator and let them sit at room temperature for about 10-15 minutes while the grill is preheating. This will help the steaks cook more evenly. Once the grill is hot, place the lamb steaks on the grill grates.

5 **Cook to Desired Doneness:** Grill the lamb leg steaks for about 4-5 minutes per side for medium-rare, or adjust the cooking time according to your preferred level of doneness. Use a meat thermometer to check the internal temperature of the steaks – it should register 145°F (63°C) for medium-rare, 160°F (71°C) for medium, or 170°F (77°C) for well-done.

6 **Rest and Serve:** Once cooked to your liking, remove the lamb leg steaks from the grill and transfer them to a cutting board. Tent the steaks loosely with foil and let them rest for about 5 minutes to allow the juices to redistribute.

7 **Slice and Serve:** After resting, slice the grilled lamb leg steaks against the grain into thin slices.

Arrange the slices on a serving platter and garnish with additional fresh herbs, if desired. Serve immediately with your choice of side dishes, such as a crisp salad or roasted vegetables.

8 **Enjoy:** Enjoy the delicious flavors of the grilled lamb leg steaks as a satisfying and wholesome meal, perfect for any occasion.

Lamb Riblets with Garlic and Herbs

These tender lamb riblets, seasoned with garlic and herbs, are slow-cooked to perfection for a melt-in-your-mouth dining experience. Enjoy them as a flavorful appetizer or main course, paired with your favorite carnivore-friendly sides.

Ingredients:

- 2 lbs. lamb riblets
- 4 cloves garlic, minced
- 2 tablespoons olive oil
- 1 tablespoon fresh rosemary, finely chopped
- 1 tablespoon fresh thyme, finely chopped
- Salt and pepper to taste

Step by Step Instructions:

1 **Prepare the Lamb Riblets:** Rinse the lamb riblets under cold water and pat them dry with paper towels. Place them in a large mixing bowl.

2 **Prepare the Marinade:** In a small bowl, combine the minced garlic, olive oil, chopped rosemary, chopped thyme, salt, and pepper. Mix well to combine.

3 **Marinate the Lamb Riblets:** Pour the marinade over the lamb riblets, ensuring they are evenly coated. Use your hands to massage the marinade into the meat. Cover the bowl with plastic wrap or transfer the riblets to a resalable plastic bag. Marinate in the refrigerator for at least 1 hour, or preferably overnight, to allow the flavors to penetrate the meat.

4 **Preheat the Oven:** Preheat your oven to 325°F (165°C).

5 **Prepare the Baking Dish:** Remove the marinated lamb riblets from the refrigerator and transfer them to a baking dish large enough to accommodate them in a single layer.

6 **Bake the Lamb Rib lets:** Cover the baking dish with aluminum foil and place it in the preheated oven. Bake for approximately 2 to 2½ hours, or until the riblets are tender and cooked through.

7 **Broil for Crispy Finish (Optional):** If desired, remove the foil during the last 10-15 minutes of baking and switch the oven to broil. Broil the riblets for an additional 5-10 minutes, or until the tops are browned and slightly crispy

8   **Serve:** Once cooked to perfection, remove the lamb riblets from the oven and let them rest for a few minutes before serving. Garnish with additional fresh herbs, if desired, and serve hot as a flavorful appetizer or main course.

9   **Enjoy:** Enjoy the tender and flavorful lamb riblets with garlic and herbs as a delicious and satisfying carnivore-friendly dish, perfect for any occasion.

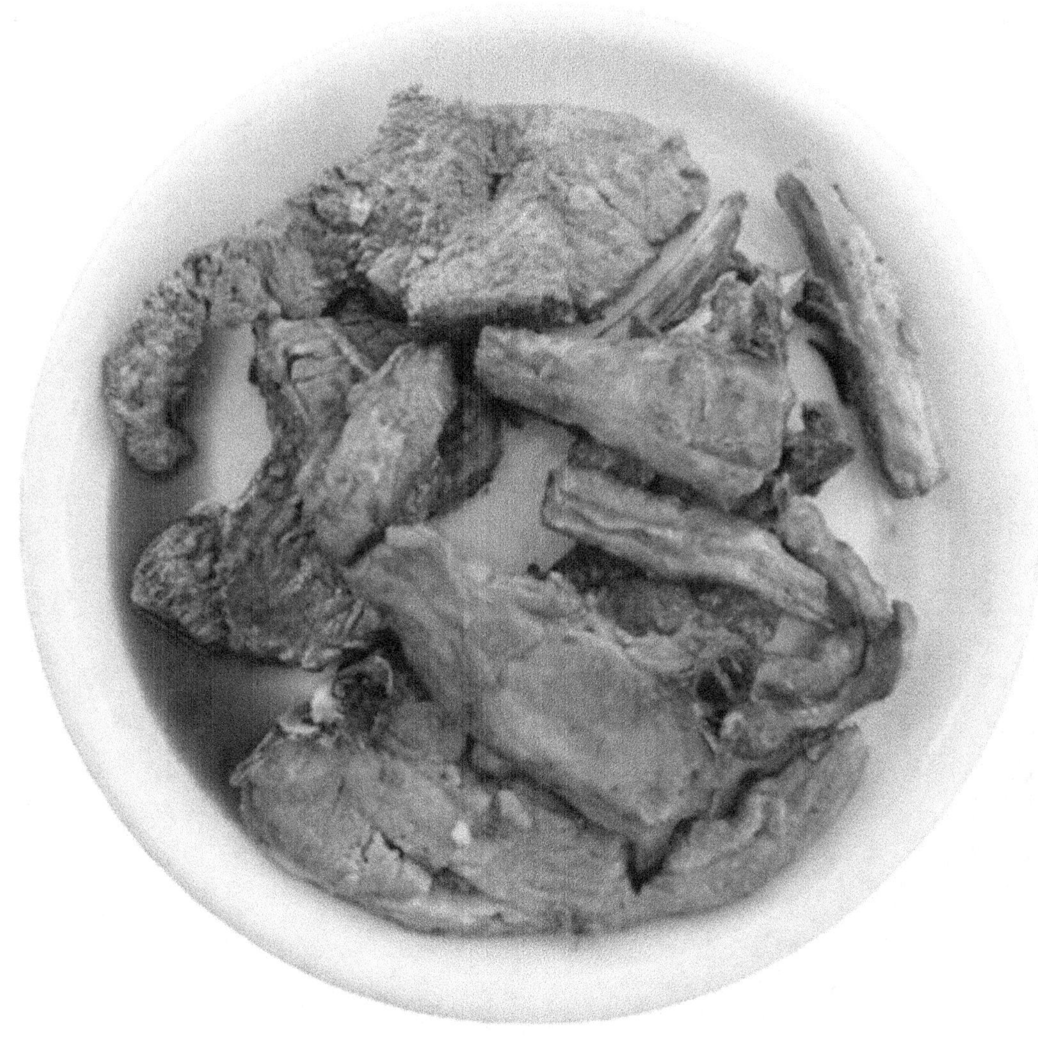

Chapter 7

SEAFOOD SENSATIONS

Seafood offers a diverse array of flavors and textures that can tantalize the taste buds of any carnivore. From succulent salmon to delicate scallops, the options are endless. In this chapter, we'll explore a variety of seafood sensations that will delight your palate and provide essential nutrients for your carnivore diet journey.

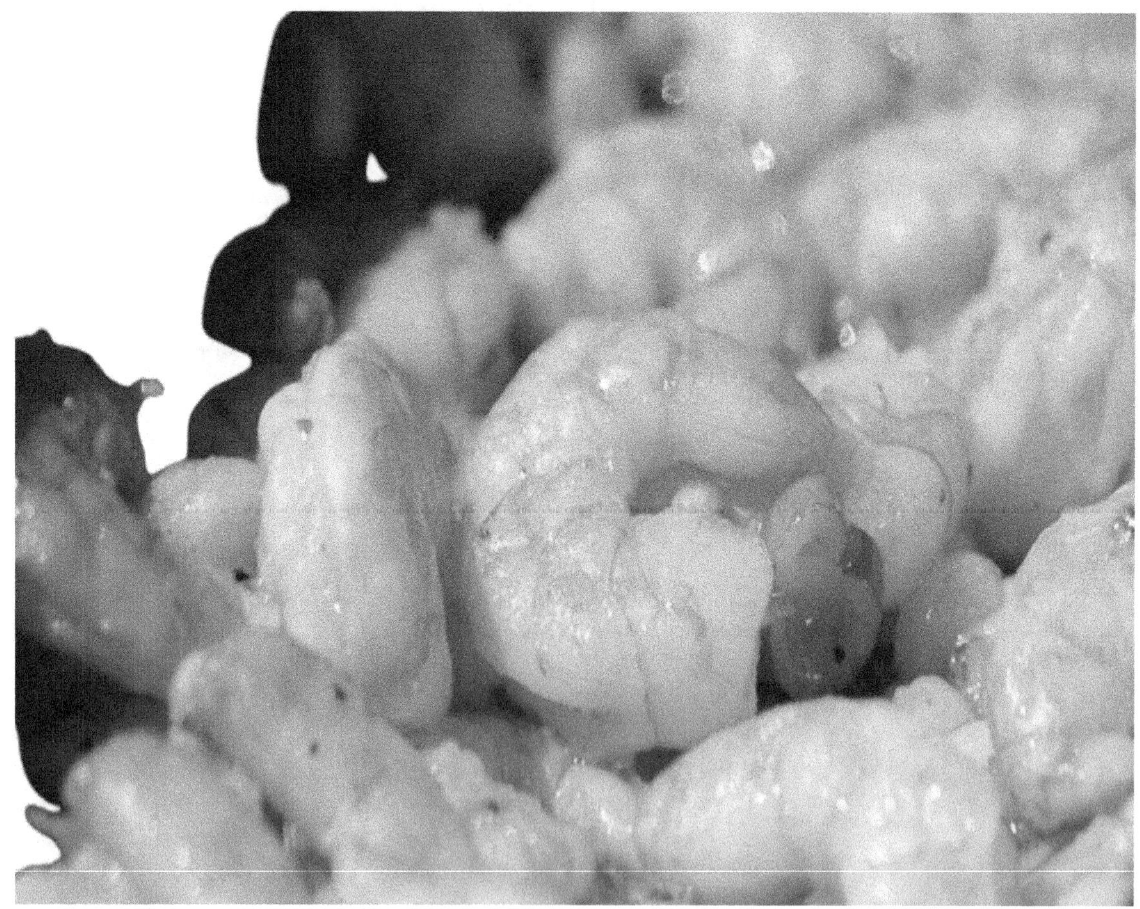

Grilled Salmon with Lemon and Herbs

Full of omega-3 fatty acids and protein, grilled salmon is a nutritious and delicious addition to your carnivore diet. The bright flavors of lemon and herbs perfectly complement the rich taste of the salmon.

Ingredients:

- 2 salmon fillets (6-8 ounces each)
- 1 lemon, sliced
- 2 tablespoons olive oil
- 2 cloves garlic, minced
- 1 teaspoon dried thyme
- 1 teaspoon dried rosemary
- Salt and pepper to taste

Step by Step Instructions:

1 Preheat your grill to medium-high heat.

2 In a small bowl, combine the olive oil, minced garlic, dried thyme, dried rosemary, salt, and pepper. Mix well to create the marinade.

3 Place the salmon fillets on a plate or in a shallow dish.

Brush the marinade over both sides of the salmon fillets, ensuring they are evenly coated.

4   Place a few lemon slices on top of each salmon fillet for added flavor.

5   Once the grill is hot, place the salmon fillets directly onto the grill grates, skin-side down.

6   Close the grill and cook the salmon for 4-5 minutes on each side, or until the flesh is opaque and flakes easily with a fork.

7   Carefully remove the grilled salmon from the grill and transfer it to a serving platter.

8   Serve the grilled salmon hot, garnished with additional lemon slices and fresh herbs if desired.

9   Enjoy your grilled salmon with lemon and herbs as a nutritious and flavorful addition to your carnivore diet!

Grilled Shrimp Skewers

Bursting with flavor and protein, grilled shrimp skewers are a quick and easy seafood option for carnivores. Simply marinate the shrimp in your favorite seasonings, thread them onto skewers, and grill until pink and slightly charred.

Ingredients:

- 1-pound large shrimp, peeled and deveined

- 2 tablespoons olive oil

- 2 cloves garlic, minced

- 1 teaspoon paprika

- 1 teaspoon dried oregano

- 1/2 teaspoon salt

- 1/4 teaspoon black pepper

- Wooden or metal skewers

Step by Step Instructions:

1 If using wooden skewers, soak them in water for at least 30 minutes to prevent them from burning on the grill.

2 In a bowl, combine the olive oil, minced garlic, paprika, dried oregano, salt, and black pepper. Mix well to create the marinade.

3 Add the peeled and deveined shrimp to the marinade, making sure they are evenly coated. Allow the shrimp to marinate for 15-20 minutes to absorb the flavors.

4 Preheat your grill to medium-high heat.

5 Thread the marinated shrimp onto the skewers, leaving a small space between each shrimp to ensure even cooking.

6 Once the grill is hot, place the shrimp skewers directly onto the grill grates.

7 Grill the shrimp skewers for 2-3 minutes on each side, or until they turn pink and slightly charred.

8 Carefully remove the grilled shrimp skewers from the grill and transfer them to a serving platter.

9 Serve the grilled shrimp skewers hot, garnished with fresh herbs or a squeeze of lemon juice if desired.

10 Enjoy your flavorful and protein-packed grilled shrimp skewers as a delicious addition to your carnivore diet!

Pan-Fried Sardines with Lemon

Sardines are a nutritional powerhouse, packed with omega-3 fatty acids, vitamin D, and protein. Pan-frying them with lemon adds a zesty freshness to these tiny fish, making them a tasty and satisfying carnivore meal.

Ingredients:

- Fresh sardines, cleaned and gutted

- Salt

- Black pepper

- Olive oil or bacon fat

- 1 lemon, sliced

- Optional: fresh herbs for garnish

Step by Step Instructions:

1 Start by cleaning and gutting the fresh sardines, if they haven't been cleaned already. Rinse them under cold water and pat them dry with paper towels.

2 Score each sardine on both sides with a sharp knife, making shallow cuts to help them cook evenly and allow the flavors to penetrate.

3 Season the sardines generously with salt and black pepper, both inside and out.

4 Heat a skillet over medium-high heat and add a drizzle of olive oil or bacon fat to coat the bottom of the pan.

5 Once the skillet is hot, carefully add the seasoned sardines to the pan, laying them in a single layer without overcrowding the pan.

6 Cook the sardines for about 3-4 minutes on each side, or until they are golden brown and crispy on the outside and cooked through.

7   During the last minute of cooking, add the sliced lemon to the skillet, allowing it to caramelize slightly and infuse the sardines with its citrusy flavor.

8   Once the sardines are cooked through and the lemon slices are caramelized, carefully remove them from the skillet and transfer them to a serving platter.

9   Garnish the pan-fried sardines with fresh herbs if desired, and serve them hot as a nutritious and flavorful carnivore meal.

10 Enjoy the deliciousness and nutritional benefits of pan-fried sardines with lemon as a satisfying addition to your carnivore diet!

Pan-Seared Cod Fillets with Lemon Butter Sauce

Cod fillets are mild in flavor and flaky in texture, making them a versatile option for carnivores. Pan-seared until golden brown and served with a tangy lemon butter sauce, they're a simple yet elegant dish that's sure to please.

Ingredients:

- 4 cod fillets, skinless and boneless
- Salt and black pepper, to taste
- 2 tablespoons olive oil or ghee
- 2 tablespoons unsalted butter
- 2 cloves garlic, minced

- Juice of 1 lemon

- 2 tablespoons chopped fresh parsley, for garnish

Step by Step Instructions:

1 Pat the cod fillets dry with paper towels and season both sides generously with salt and black pepper.

2 Heat a large skillet over medium-high heat and add olive oil or ghee to the pan, swirling to coat the bottom evenly.

3 Once the skillet is hot, carefully add the seasoned cod fillets to the pan, making sure not to overcrowd them. Cook in batches if necessary.

4 Sear the cod fillets for about 4-5 minutes on each side, or until they are golden brown and cooked through. The flesh should be opaque and flake easily with a fork.

5 While the cod is cooking, prepare the lemon butter sauce. In a small saucepan, melt the butter over medium heat. Add the minced garlic and cook for 1-2 minutes, or until fragrant.

6 Remove the saucepan from the heat and stir in the lemon juice. Season the sauce with salt and pepper to taste, adjusting the flavors as needed.

7 Once the cod fillets are done cooking, transfer them to a serving platter or individual plates.

8 Drizzle the lemon butter sauce over the cooked cod fillets, ensuring each fillet is generously coated with the sauce.

9 Garnish the cod fillets with chopped fresh parsley for a pop of color and freshness.

10 Serve the pan-seared cod fillets with lemon butter sauce immediately, accompanied by your favorite carnivore-friendly sides.

11 Enjoy the delightful flavors of tender cod paired with tangy lemon butter sauce as a satisfying and elegant addition to your carnivore diet!

Grilled Octopus Tentacles

Grilled octopus' tentacles are a delicacy that offers a unique texture and flavor experience. Marinated in olive oil, lemon, and herbs, then grilled to perfection, they're tender on the inside and crispy on the outside, making them a true seafood sensation.

Ingredients:

- 2-3 octopus' tentacles, cleaned and thawed if frozen
- 1/4 cup olive oil
- Juice of 1 lemon
- 2 cloves garlic, minced
- 1 teaspoon dried oregano
- Salt and black pepper, to taste

- Lemon wedges, for serving

- Chopped fresh parsley, for garnish

Step by Step Instructions:

1 Preheat your grill to medium-high heat (about 400°F to 450°F or 200°C to 230°C).

2 In a small bowl, whisk together the olive oil, lemon juice, minced garlic, dried oregano, salt, and black pepper to create the marinade.

3 Place the cleaned octopus' tentacles in a shallow dish or resalable plastic bag. Pour the marinade over the tentacles, ensuring they are evenly coated. Allow the octopus to marinate for at least 30 minutes to 1 hour in the refrigerator, turning occasionally to coat.

4 Once the octopus has finished marinating, remove it from the refrigerator and let it come to room temperature for about 10-15 minutes before grilling.

5 Carefully oil the grill grates to prevent sticking. Place the octopus' tentacles on the grill and cook for about 3-4 minutes per side, or until they are charred and crispy on the outside and tender on the inside. Be cautious not to overcook, as octopus can become tough if cooked for too long.

6 Once grilled to perfection, remove the octopus' tentacles from the grill and transfer them to a serving platter.

7   Garnish the grilled octopus' tentacles with chopped fresh parsley and serve hot with lemon wedges on the side for squeezing over the octopus.

8   Enjoy the irresistible flavors and textures of grilled octopus' tentacles as a delightful addition to your carnivore-friendly seafood feast!

Seared Scallops with Butter and Garlic

Seared scallops are a gourmet treat that's surprisingly easy to prepare. Sautéed in butter and garlic until golden brown and caramelized, they're sweet, succulent, and perfect for a carnivore-friendly meal.

Ingredients:

- 1 pound fresh scallops, patted dry with paper towels
- 2 tablespoons unsalted butter
- 2 cloves garlic, minced
- Salt and black pepper, to taste
- Fresh lemon wedges, for serving
- Chopped fresh parsley, for garnish (optional)

Step by Step Instructions:

1   **Prepare the Scallops:**

- Pat the scallops dry with paper towels to remove any excess moisture. This will help achieve a nice sear.

- Season both sides of the scallops with salt and black pepper to taste.

2   Heat the Pan:

- Heat a large skillet or frying pan over medium-high heat. Ensure the pan is hot before adding the scallops.

3   Sear the Scallops:

- Add the butter to the hot pan and swirl it around to coat the bottom evenly.

- Once the butter is melted and sizzling, carefully add the seasoned scallops to the pan in a single layer, making sure they are not overcrowded.

- Let the scallops cook undisturbed for about 2-3 minutes, or until a golden crust forms on the bottom. Avoid moving or flipping the scallops too early to ensure a proper sear.

- Using a pair of tongs, flip the scallops over and continue cooking for another 2-3 minutes, or until the other side is also golden brown and caramelized. The scallops should be opaque and firm to the touch but still slightly translucent in the center.

4   Add Garlic:

- Add the minced garlic to the pan with the scallops during the last minute of cooking.

- Stir the garlic around the pan and allow it to become fragrant, infusing the scallops with its flavor.

5 Serve:

- Transfer the seared scallops to a serving platter or individual plates.

- Garnish with chopped fresh parsley, if desired, for a pop of color and freshness.

- Serve the seared scallops hot with fresh lemon wedges on the side for squeezing over the scallops just before eating.

6 Enjoy:

- Dive into the succulent and flavorful seared scallops, savoring the delicate sweetness and buttery richness with each bite.

Bacon-Wrapped Scallops

Elevate your scallop game by wrapping them in crispy bacon before searing. The combination of sweet scallops and salty bacon creates a mouthwatering contrast of flavors and textures that's sure to impress.

Ingredients:

- 1 pound fresh scallops, patted dry with paper towels
- 8-10 slices of bacon, cut in half crosswise
- Salt and black pepper, to taste

- Toothpicks or small skewers

Step by Step Instructions:

1 **Prepare the Scallops:**
   - Pat the scallops dry with paper towels to remove any excess moisture.
   - Season both sides of the scallops with salt and black pepper to taste.

2 **Wrap the Scallops with Bacon:**
- Take a half-slice of bacon and wrap it around each scallop, securing it in place with a toothpick or small skewer. Repeat for all the scallops.

3 **Sear the Bacon-Wrapped Scallops:**
- Heat a large skillet or frying pan over medium-high heat.

- Once the pan is hot, carefully add the bacon-wrapped scallops to the pan in a single layer, making sure they are not overcrowded.

- Let the scallops cook undisturbed for about 2-3 minutes, or until the bacon on the bottom is crispy and golden brown.

- Using a pair of tongs, carefully flip the scallops over and cook for another 2-3 minutes, or until the bacon on the other side is also crispy and golden brown. The scallops should be opaque and firm to the touch but still slightly translucent in the center.

4 **Serve:**

- Transfer the bacon-wrapped scallops to a serving platter or individual plates.

- Remove the toothpicks or skewers before serving.

- Serve the bacon-wrapped scallops hot as an appetizer or main course, garnished with fresh herbs or a squeeze of lemon juice if desired.

Enjoy:

- Enjoy the irresistible combination of sweet, tender scallops and crispy, savory bacon with each delicious bite.

Smoked Salmon Bites

Smoked salmon is a versatile ingredient that can be enjoyed on its own or incorporated into a variety of dishes. These smoked salmon bites are perfect for snacking or serving as an elegant appetizer at your next gathering.

Ingredients:

- ounces smoked salmon, thinly sliced
- ounces' cream cheese, softened
- 2 tablespoons fresh dill, chopped
- 1 tablespoon capers, drained
- 1 tablespoon red onion, finely chopped
- Lemon wedges, for serving

- Crackers or cucumber slices, for serving (optional)

Step by Step Instructions:

1 Prepare the Cream Cheese Mixture:

- In a small mixing bowl, combine the softened cream cheese, chopped fresh dill, drained capers, and finely chopped red onion. Mix well until all the ingredients are evenly incorporated.

2 Assemble the Smoked Salmon Bites:

- Lay out the thinly sliced smoked salmon on a clean work surface.

- Take a small spoonful of the cream cheese mixture and spread it evenly onto each slice of smoked salmon.

- Roll up each slice of smoked salmon into a tight cylinder, enclosing the cream cheese mixture inside.

3 Chill the Smoked Salmon Bites:

- Place the rolled-up smoked salmon bites on a serving platter or plate.

- Cover the plate with plastic wrap and refrigerate for at least 30 minutes to allow the flavors to meld and the cream cheese mixture to set.

Serve:

- Once chilled, remove the smoked salmon bites from the refrigerator.

- Arrange them on a serving platter and garnish with additional fresh dill or capers if desired.

- Serve the smoked salmon bites with lemon wedges on the side for squeezing over the top.

- Optionally, serve the smoked salmon bites with crackers or cucumber slices for a low-carb alternative.

Enjoy:

- Enjoy these delicious smoked salmon bites as a flavorful snack or elegant appetizer, perfect for any occasion.

Tuna Salad with Mayonnaise and Celery

Tuna salad is a classic dish that's simple to prepare and bursting with flavor. Mix canned tuna with mayonnaise, celery, and your favorite seasonings for a quick and satisfying meal that's perfect for lunch or dinner.

Ingredients:

- 2 cans (5 ounces each) of tuna, drained
- 1/4 cup mayonnaise
- 1/4 cup celery, finely chopped
- 1 tablespoon lemon juice

- 1 teaspoon Dijon mustard (optional)

- Salt and pepper to taste

- Lettuce leaves or low-carb wraps, for serving (optional)

Step by Step Instructions:

1 **Prepare the Tuna Salad:**

- In a mixing bowl, add the drained tuna.

- Add the mayonnaise, finely chopped celery, lemon juice, and Dijon mustard (if using) to the tuna.

2 **Mix the Ingredients:**

- Using a fork or spoon, mix all the ingredients together until well combined and the tuna is evenly coated with the mayonnaise mixture.

- Taste the tuna salad and adjust the seasoning with salt and pepper according to your preference.

3 **Chill (Optional):**

- If time allows and for enhanced flavor, cover the bowl with plastic wrap and refrigerate the tuna salad for about 30 minutes to 1 hour to allow the flavors to meld together.

4 **Serve:**

- Once chilled (if desired), remove the tuna salad from the refrigerator.

- Serve the tuna salad on a bed of lettuce leaves for a low-carb option, or use it as a filling for low-carb wraps or sandwiches if preferred.

5 **Enjoy:** Enjoy the tuna salad as a quick and satisfying meal for lunch or dinner, or as a tasty snack served with your favorite low-carb accompaniments.

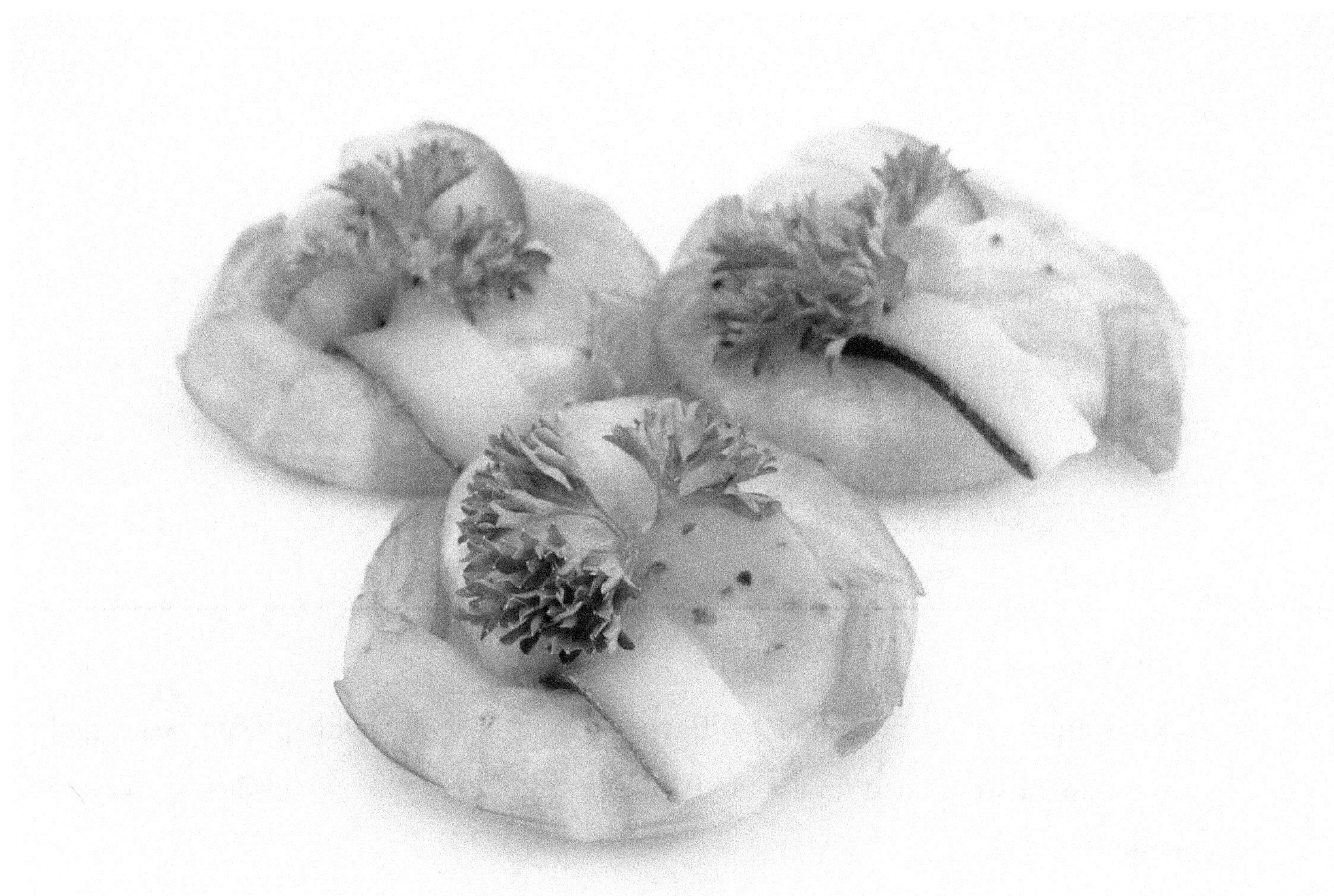

Chapter 8

MISCELLANEOUS MEAT MARVELS

In this chapter, we explore a variety of carnivore-friendly recipes featuring unique meats such as bison, venison, duck, rabbit, and more. These recipes offer diverse flavors and textures to keep your carnivore diet exciting and satisfying.

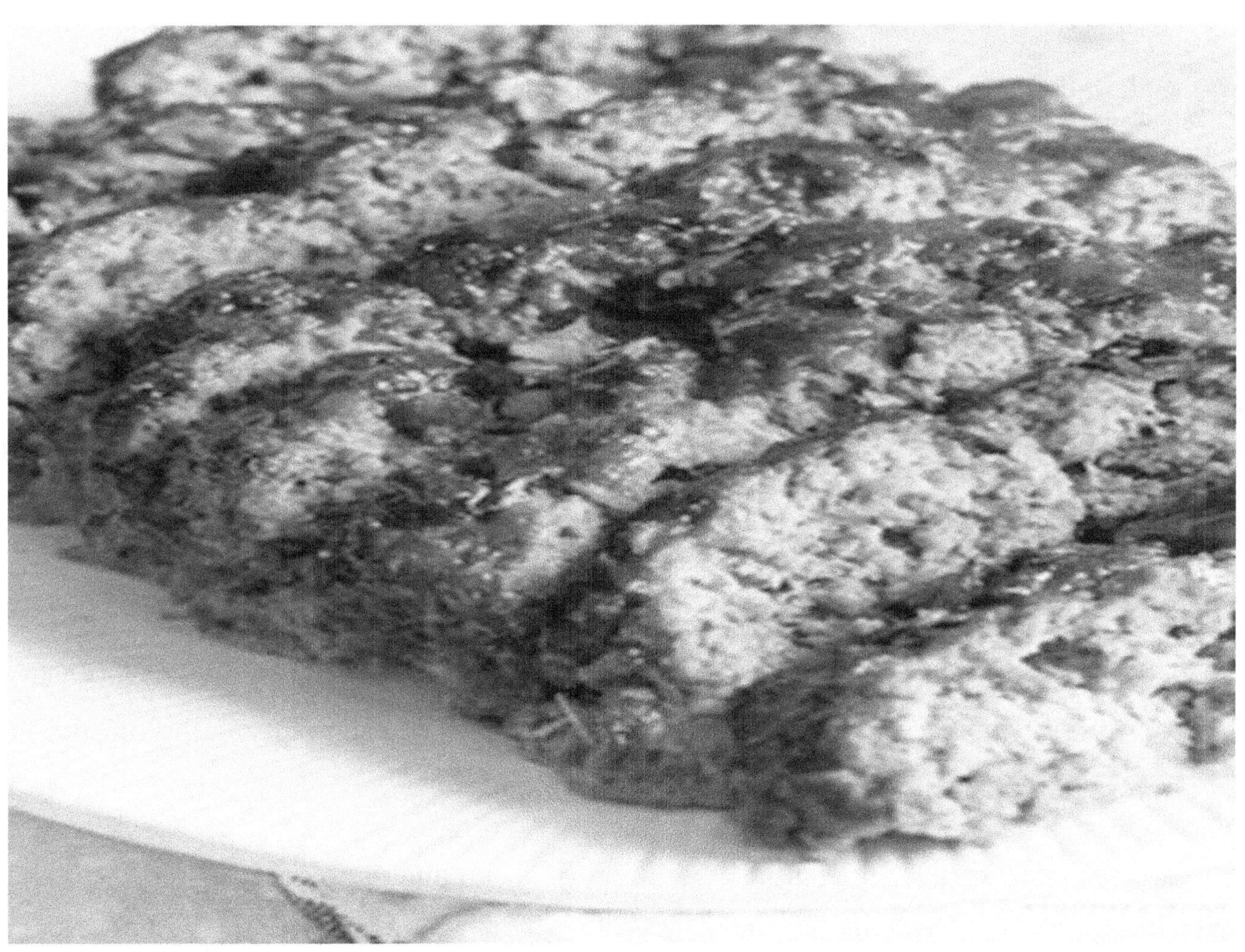

Full of flavor and healthy fats, bison burgers paired with creamy avocado create a delicious and satisfying meal.

Ingredients:

- 1 lb. ground bison meat
- 1 ripe avocado
- Salt and pepper, to taste
- Optional toppings: lettuce, tomato, onion, cheese (if desired)
- Optional condiments: mustard, mayonnaise, ketchup

Step by Step Instructions:

1 Prepare the Bison Patties:

- In a mixing bowl, gently combine the ground bison meat with salt and pepper. Be careful not to overwork the meat to maintain its tenderness.

- Divide the seasoned meat into equal portions and shape them into burger patties of desired thickness. Make an indentation in the center of each patty with your thumb to prevent them from puffing up during cooking.

- Season both sides of the patties with additional salt and pepper, if desired.

2 Cook the Bison Patties:

- Preheat a grill or skillet over medium-high heat. If using a skillet, add a small amount of cooking oil to prevent sticking.

- Once the grill or skillet is hot, add the bison patties and cook for about 4-5 minutes on each side, or until they reach your preferred level of doneness. Bison meat is lean, so take care not to overcook to avoid dryness. For medium-rare burgers, aim for an internal temperature of about 145°F (63°C), while medium is around 160°F (71°C).

3 Prepare the Avocado:

- While the burgers are cooking, slice the ripe avocado and remove the pit. Scoop out the flesh and slice it into thin pieces.

4 Assemble the Burgers:

- Once the bison patties are cooked to your liking, remove them from the grill or skillet and let them rest for a few minutes.

- To assemble the burgers, place a cooked bison patty on a plate or bun, then top it with sliced avocado and any desired toppings or condiments.

- Serve the bison burgers immediately, either on their own or with your favorite side dishes.

5 Enjoy:

- Indulge in the delicious flavors of the bison burgers with creamy avocado, and savor each bite of this satisfying and nutritious meal.

Storage:

- Store any leftover cooked bison burgers in an airtight container in the refrigerator for up to 3-4 days. Reheat before serving, if desired.

Venison Stew with Mushrooms

Tender chunks of venison simmered with mushrooms in a rich broth make for a hearty and comforting stew.

Ingredients:

- 2 lbs. venison stew meat, cubed
- oz. mushrooms, sliced
- 1 onion, chopped
- cloves garlic, minced
- cups beef broth
- 1 cup red wine (optional)
- 2 tablespoons tomato paste
- 2 bay leaves
- 1 teaspoon dried thyme
- 1 teaspoon dried rosemary
- Salt and pepper to taste
- 2 tablespoons olive oil

Step-by-Step Instructions:

1 **Prepare the Venison:** Season the cubed venison stew meat with salt and pepper to taste.

2 **Sear the Venison:** In a large pot or Dutch oven, heat 1 tablespoon of olive oil over medium-high heat. Add the seasoned venison cubes in batches and sear on all sides until browned. Remove the seared venison from the pot and set aside.

3 **Sauté the Aromatics:** In the same pot, add another tablespoon of olive oil if needed. Add the chopped onion and minced garlic, and sauté until softened and fragrant.

4 **Add the Mushrooms:** Add the sliced mushrooms to the pot and cook until they begin to brown and release their juices.

5 **Deglaze the Pot:** Pour in the red wine (if using) to deglaze the pot, scraping up any browned bits from the bottom for added flavor.

6 **Simmer with Broth:** Return the seared venison to the pot. Pour in the beef broth and add the tomato paste, bay leaves, dried thyme, and dried rosemary. Stir to combine.

7 **Simmer:** Bring the stew to a boil, then reduce the heat to low. Cover and simmer for 2-3 hours, or until the venison is tender and the flavors have melded together.

8 **Adjust Seasoning:** Taste the stew and adjust the seasoning with salt and pepper if needed.

9 Serve: Remove the bay leaves before serving. Ladle the venison stew into bowls and garnish with fresh herbs if desired. Serve hot and enjoy this hearty and comforting dish.

This venison stew with mushrooms is perfect for warming up on a cold day, and the tender chunks of venison combined with earthy mushrooms create a flavorful and satisfying meal.

Duck Breast with Orange Glaze

Succulent duck breast drizzled with a tangy orange glaze offers a delightful combination of flavors that's both elegant and delicious.

Ingredients:

- 2 duck breasts, skin-on
- Salt and pepper to taste
- 1 tablespoon olive oil
- 2 cloves garlic, minced
- 1/2 cup orange juice
- 2 tablespoons honey
- Zest of 1 orange
- 2 tablespoons balsamic vinegar
- 1 tablespoon soy sauce
- 1 teaspoon grated ginger

- Fresh parsley or green onions for garnish (optional)

Step-by-Step Instructions:

1. **Prepare the Duck Breast:** Pat the duck breasts dry with paper towels. Score the skin of each duck breast in a crosshatch pattern, being careful not to cut into the meat. Season both sides of the duck breasts with salt and pepper.

2. **Sear the Duck Breast:** Heat a skillet over medium-high heat. Once hot, add the duck breasts skin-side down. Cook for about 5-7 minutes, or until the skin is crispy and golden brown. Flip the duck breasts and cook for an additional 2-3 minutes on the other side. Remove the duck breasts from the skillet and set aside.

3. **Make the Orange Glaze:** In the same skillet, reduce the heat to medium. Add the minced garlic and sauté for about 30 seconds until fragrant. Pour in the orange juice, honey, orange zest, balsamic vinegar, soy sauce, and grated ginger. Stir well to combine.

4. **Simmer the Glaze:** Allow the glaze to simmer and reduce for about 5-7 minutes, or until it thickens slightly and coats the back of a spoon.

5. **Glaze the Duck Breast:** Return the duck breasts to the skillet, skin-side up, and spoon the orange glaze over them. Cook for an additional 2-3 minutes, basting the duck breasts with the glaze.

6   **Rest and Slice:** Remove the duck breasts from the skillet and let them rest for a few minutes before slicing them thinly against the grain.

7   **Serve:** Arrange the sliced duck breast on a serving platter, drizzle with any remaining glaze from the skillet, and garnish with fresh parsley or green onions if desired. Serve hot and enjoy this elegant and flavorful dish.

This duck breast with orange glaze is a sophisticated yet easy-to-make dish that's perfect for a special dinner at home. The crispy skin and tender meat paired with the tangy and sweet orange glaze create a memorable flavor experience.

Rabbit Stew with Thyme

Rabbit stew seasoned with fragrant thyme is a wholesome and nourishing dish that's perfect for colder days.

Ingredients:

- 1 whole rabbit, cut into pieces
- Salt and pepper to taste
- 2 tablespoons olive oil
- 1 onion, diced
- 2 carrots, diced
- 2 celery stalks, diced

- cloves garlic, minced

- 2 cups chicken or beef broth

- 1 cup dry white wine (optional)

- 2 bay leaves

- 2 sprigs fresh thyme

- 1 teaspoon dried thyme

- 1 tablespoon tomato paste

- 2 tablespoons all-purpose flour (optional, for thickening)

- Chopped fresh parsley for garnish (optional)

Step-by-Step Instructions:

1 **Prepare the Rabbit:** Rinse the rabbit pieces under cold water and pat them dry with paper towels. Season generously with salt and pepper on all sides.

2 **Brown the Rabbit:** Heat the olive oil in a large Dutch oven or heavy-bottomed pot over medium-high heat. Add the rabbit pieces in batches and brown them on all sides, about 2-3 minutes per side. Remove the browned rabbit pieces and set aside.

3 **Sauté the Vegetables:** In the same pot, add the diced onion, carrots, and celery. Sauté for 5-7 minutes, or until the vegetables are softened and lightly browned. Add the minced garlic and cook for an additional 1-2 minutes.

4 **Deglaze the Pot:** Pour in the chicken or beef broth and white wine (if using), scraping the bottom of the pot with a wooden spoon to loosen any browned bits stuck to the bottom.

5 **Add the Rabbit and Herbs:** Return the browned rabbit pieces to the pot. Add the bay leaves, fresh thyme sprigs, dried thyme, and tomato paste. Stir to combine.

6 **Simmer the Stew:** Bring the stew to a simmer, then reduce the heat to low. Cover the pot and let the stew simmer gently for 1.5 to 2 hours, or until the rabbit is tender and easily pulls away from the bone.

7 **Thicken the Stew (Optional):** If desired, you can thicken the stew by mixing 2 tablespoons of all-purpose flour with a little water to form a slurry. Stir the slurry into the stew and simmer for an additional 10-15 minutes until thickened.

8 **Adjust Seasoning:** Taste the stew and adjust the seasoning with salt and pepper if needed.

9 **Serve:** Ladle the rabbit stew into bowls, garnish with chopped fresh parsley if desired, and serve hot. Enjoy this hearty and flavorful rabbit stew with thyme on a chilly day for a comforting meal.

Bison Chili with Diced Tomatoes and Spices

Bison chili, made with diced tomatoes and a blend of spices, is a hearty and flavorful option for carnivores craving a classic comfort food.

Ingredients:

- 1 lb. ground bison meat
- 1 onion, diced
- cloves garlic, minced
- 1 bell pepper, diced
- 1 can (14.5 oz.) diced tomatoes
- 2 tablespoons tomato paste
- 2 cups beef broth
- 1 can (15 oz.) kidney beans, drained and rinsed (optional)
- 2 tablespoons chili powder
- 1 teaspoon ground cumin
- 1 teaspoon paprika
- 1/2 teaspoon ground coriander
- 1/2 teaspoon dried oregano
- Salt and pepper to taste
- Olive oil for cooking
- Optional toppings: shredded cheese, sour cream, chopped green onions, sliced jalapeños

Step-by-Step Instructions:

1. **Sauté the Aromatics:** Heat a drizzle of olive oil in a large pot or Dutch oven over medium heat.

Add the diced onion, minced garlic, and diced bell pepper. Sauté for 5-7 minutes, or until the vegetables are softened and translucent.

2 **Brown the Bison:** Push the sautéed vegetables to the side of the pot and add the ground bison meat. Break up the meat with a spatula and cook until browned, about 5-7 minutes.

3 **Add Tomatoes and Tomato Paste:** Stir in the diced tomatoes and tomato paste, scraping up any browned bits from the bottom of the pot.

4 **Season the Chili:** Add the chili powder, ground cumin, paprika, ground coriander, dried oregano, salt, and pepper to the pot. Stir well to combine and coat the meat and vegetables with the spices.

5 **Simmer the Chili:** Pour in the beef broth and bring the chili to a simmer. Reduce the heat to low and let it simmer, uncovered, for about 30-40 minutes, stirring occasionally.

6 **Add Beans (Optional):** If using kidney beans, add them to the chili during the last 10 minutes of cooking. This step is optional and can be omitted for a bean-free chili.

7 **Adjust Seasoning:** Taste the chili and adjust the seasoning with salt and pepper if needed. You can also adjust the spice level by adding more chili powder or paprika if desired.

8 Serve: Ladle the bison chili into bowls and serve hot. Garnish with your favorite toppings such as shredded cheese, sour cream, chopped green onions, or sliced jalapeños. Enjoy this hearty and flavorful bison chili with diced tomatoes and spices for a satisfying carnivore meal.

Bison Ribeye Steak with Garlic Aioli

Juicy bison ribeye steak served with creamy garlic aioli is a decadent carnivore meal that's sure to impress.

Ingredients:

- 2 bison ribeye steaks, about 1 inch thick
- Salt and black pepper to taste
- Olive oil for cooking
- Fresh parsley or chives for garnish (optional)

For the Garlic Aioli:

- 1/2 cup mayonnaise
- 2 cloves garlic, minced
- 1 tablespoon lemon juice
- Salt and black pepper to taste

Step-by-Step Instructions:

1. **Prepare the Garlic Aioli:**

- In a small bowl, combine the mayonnaise, minced garlic, and lemon juice. Stir well to combine.
- Season the aioli with salt and black pepper to taste. Cover and refrigerate until ready to serve.

2. **Preheat the Grill or Skillet:**

- Preheat your grill or a cast-iron skillet over medium-high heat. Brush the grill grates or skillet with olive oil to prevent sticking.

3. **Season the Steaks:**

- Pat the bison ribeye steaks dry with paper towels to remove any excess moisture.
- Season both sides of the steaks generously with salt and black pepper.

4. **Grill or Sear the Steaks:**

- Place the seasoned steaks on the preheated grill or skillet. Cook for about 4-5 minutes on each side for medium-rare, or adjust the cooking time according to your desired level of doneness.

- For grill marks, rotate the steaks halfway through cooking on each side.

5. Rest the Steaks:

- Once cooked to your liking, transfer the steaks to a cutting board and let them rest for 5-10 minutes. This allows the juices to redistribute, ensuring a juicy and tender steak.

6. Serve with Garlic Aioli:

- Slice the rested bison ribeye steaks against the grain into thick slices.

- Arrange the sliced steaks on a serving platter and drizzle with the prepared garlic aioli.

- Garnish with fresh parsley or chives if desired.

- Serve immediately and enjoy the juicy bison ribeye steak with creamy garlic aioli for a decadent carnivore meal that's sure to impress.

Bison Meatloaf with Tomato Sauce

Bison meatloaf topped with tangy tomato sauce is a comforting and satisfying dish that's perfect for family dinners.

Ingredients:

For the Meatloaf:

- 1 lb. ground bison

- 1 onion, finely chopped

- 2 cloves garlic, minced

- 1/2 cup almond flour (or breadcrumbs)

- 1 egg

- 1 teaspoon salt

- 1/2 teaspoon black pepper

- 1 teaspoon dried thyme

- 1 teaspoon dried oregano

- 1/2 teaspoon smoked paprika

- 2 tablespoons tomato paste

For the Tomato Sauce:

- 1 cup crushed tomatoes

- 2 tablespoons tomato paste

- 1 tablespoon apple cider vinegar

- 1 tablespoon olive oil

- 1 teaspoon dried basil

- 1 teaspoon dried oregano

- Salt and black pepper to taste

Step-by-Step Instructions:

1. Preheat the Oven:

- Preheat your oven to 375°F (190°C). Grease a loaf pan with olive oil or line it with parchment paper.

2. Prepare the Meatloaf Mixture:

- In a large mixing bowl, combine the ground bison, finely chopped onion, minced garlic, almond flour, egg, salt, black pepper, dried thyme, dried oregano, smoked paprika, and tomato paste.

- Mix the ingredients together until well combined. Be careful not to overmix.

3. Shape the Meatloaf:

- Transfer the meatloaf mixture to the prepared loaf pan. Use your hands to shape it into a loaf shape, pressing it firmly into the pan.

4. Prepare the Tomato Sauce:

- In a small bowl, combine the crushed tomatoes, tomato paste, apple cider vinegar, olive oil, dried basil, dried oregano, salt, and black pepper. Stir well to combine.

5. Top the Meatloaf with Tomato Sauce:

- Spread the prepared tomato sauce evenly over the top of the meatloaf, covering it completely.

6. Bake the Meatloaf:

- Place the meatloaf in the preheated oven and bake for 45-55 minutes, or until the internal temperature reaches 160°F (71°C) and the top is golden brown.

7. Rest and Serve:

- Once cooked, remove the meatloaf from the oven and let it rest for 10-15 minutes before slicing.
- Slice the bison meatloaf into thick slices and serve warm with your favorite side dishes.

8. Enjoy:

- Serve the bison meatloaf with tomato sauce for a comforting and satisfying carnivore-friendly meal that's perfect for family dinners.

Bison Liver Sautéed in Butter

Nutrient-dense bison liver sautéed in butter is a flavorful and nourishing option for carnivores looking to incorporate organ meats into their diet.

Ingredients:

- 1 lb. bison liver, sliced
- tablespoons butter
- Salt and pepper to taste
- Optional: minced garlic or onions for additional flavor

Step-by-Step Instructions:

1. Prepare the Bison Liver:

- Rinse the bison liver slices under cold water and pat them dry with paper towels. Remove any membranes or connective tissue if necessary.

2. Season the Liver:

- Season the bison liver slices with salt and pepper to taste. You can also add minced garlic or onions for additional flavor, if desired. Allow the liver to marinate for a few minutes while you prepare the skillet.

3. Heat the Skillet:

- Heat a skillet or frying pan over medium heat. Add the butter and allow it to melt and coat the bottom of the skillet evenly.

4. Sauté the Bison Liver:

- Once the butter is hot and bubbling, carefully add the seasoned bison liver slices to the skillet in a single layer. Be careful not to overcrowd the skillet, as this can prevent proper browning.

- Sauté the bison liver slices for 2-3 minutes on each side, or until they are cooked through and nicely browned on the outside. The cooking time may vary depending on the thickness of the liver slices and your desired level of doneness.

5. Check for Doneness:

- To ensure that the bison liver is cooked to your liking, you can use a meat thermometer to check the internal temperature. The USDA recommends cooking liver to an internal temperature of 160°F (71°C).

6. Serve Warm:

- Once the bison liver is cooked to your desired doneness, remove it from the skillet and transfer it to a serving plate. Serve the sautéed bison liver immediately while it is still warm.

7. Enjoy:

- Enjoy the flavorful and nutrient-dense bison liver sautéed in butter as a delicious and nourishing option for your carnivore diet. Serve it alongside your favorite side dishes or enjoy it on its own for a satisfying meal.

Bison Tongue Skewers

Grilled bison tongue skewers offer a unique and delicious way to enjoy this underrated cut of meat, packed with flavor and nutrients.

Ingredients:

- 1 bison tongue
- Salt and pepper to taste
- Wooden skewers, soaked in water for at least 30 minutes

Step-by-Step Instructions:

1. Prepare the Bison Tongue:

- Rinse the bison tongue under cold water and pat it dry with paper towels. Trim off any excess fat or membrane from the surface of the tongue.

2. Tenderize and Season the Tongue:

- Place the bison tongue in a large pot and cover it with water. Add salt and pepper to taste, and any additional seasonings of your choice, such as garlic or herbs.

- Bring the water to a boil, then reduce the heat to low and simmer the bison tongue for approximately 2-3 hours, or until it is tender and easily pierced with a fork.

3. Remove the Tongue and Cool:

- Once the bison tongue is tender, remove it from the pot and place it in a bowl of cold water to cool slightly. This will make it easier to handle and peel.

4. Peel the Tongue:

- Use a sharp knife to peel off the tough outer layer of skin from the bison tongue. You can also use your fingers to peel away any remaining skin or membrane.

5. Slice the Tongue:

- Once the bison tongue is peeled, slice it into thin strips or cubes, depending on your preference. Thread the slices onto wooden skewers, leaving some space between each piece to ensure even cooking.

6. Grill the Skewers:

- Preheat your grill to medium-high heat.

Place the bison tongue skewers on the grill and cook for 2-3 minutes on each side, or until they are nicely charred and heated through.

7. Serve Warm:

- Once the bison tongue skewers are grilled to perfection, remove them from the grill and transfer them to a serving platter. Serve the skewers warm as a unique and flavorful appetizer or main course.

8. Enjoy:

- Enjoy the delicious and nutrient-rich grilled bison tongue skewers with your favorite dipping sauce or side dishes. These skewers are sure to be a hit at your next barbecue or gathering!
- Each of these recipes provides a unique and delicious way to enjoy a variety of meats, offering a diverse range of flavors and textures to keep your carnivore diet exciting and satisfying.

Whether you're craving a comforting stew, a gourmet steak, or a nutrient-packed organ meat, these miscellaneous meat marvels have got you covered.

Chapter 9

SIDE DISHES AND EXTRAS

In this chapter, we'll explore a variety of side dishes and extras that complement carnivore meals, adding flavor, texture, and nutrition to your plate.

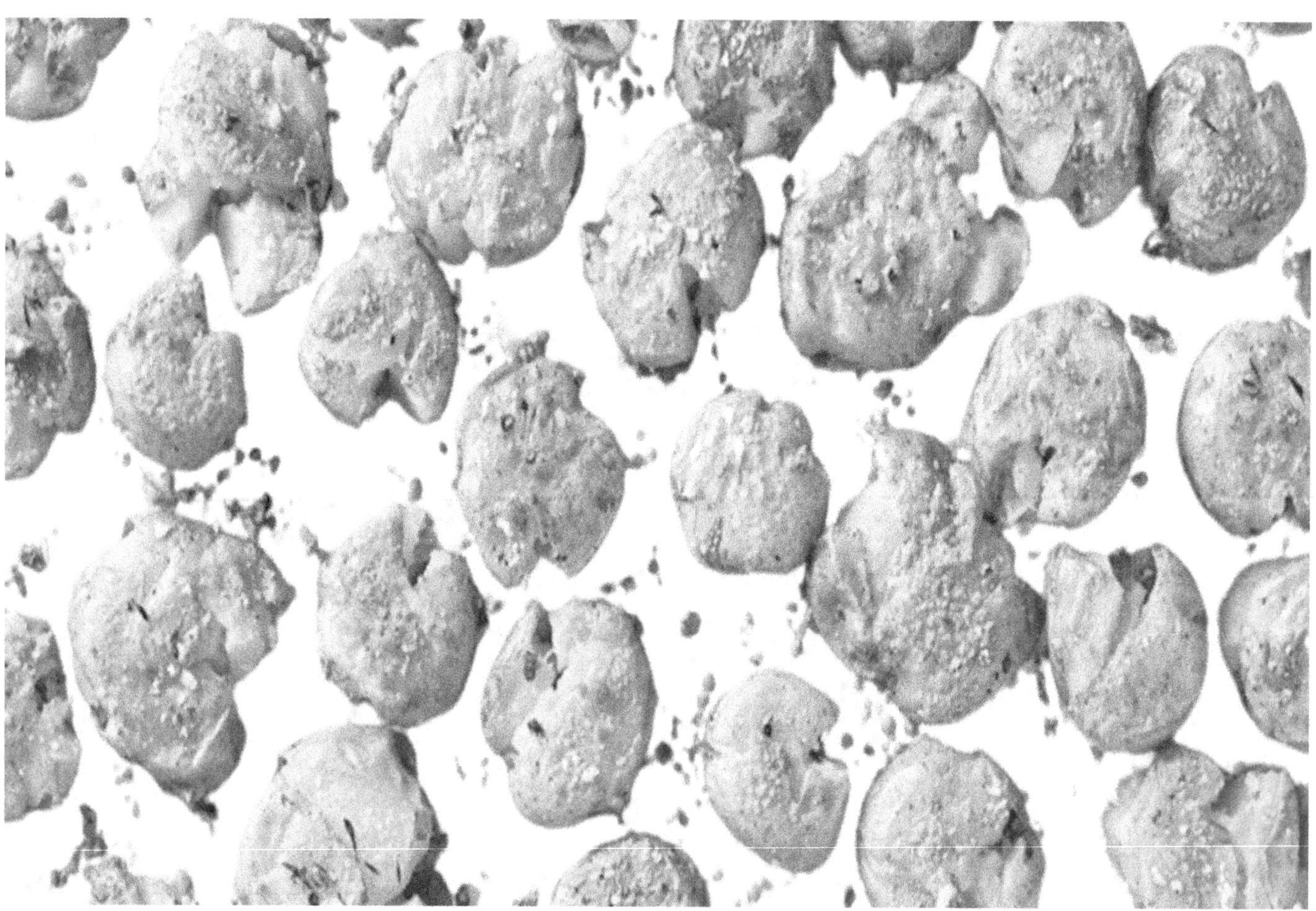

Bacon-Wrapped Asparagus Spears

Asparagus spears wrapped in crispy bacon are a savory and satisfying side dish that pairs perfectly with any carnivore meal.

Ingredients:

- Fresh asparagus spears
- Thinly sliced bacon strips (one strip per asparagus spear)
- Olive oil (optional)
- Salt and pepper to taste

Step by Step Instructions:

1. **Preheat the Oven:** Preheat your oven to 400°F (200°C).

2. **Prepare the Asparagus:** Wash the asparagus spears thoroughly and trim off the tough ends. If the spears are thick, you may want to peel the bottom portion to ensure tenderness.

3. **Wrap with Bacon:** Take one slice of bacon and wrap it around each asparagus spear, starting from the bottom and working your way up to the top. Ensure that the bacon is tightly wrapped around the asparagus to prevent it from unraveling during cooking.

4. **Season:** If desired, lightly drizzle the bacon-wrapped asparagus spears with olive oil for extra flavor and to help with browning. Season with salt and pepper to taste.

5. **Arrange on Baking Sheet:** Place the bacon-wrapped asparagus spears on a baking sheet in a single layer, ensuring that they are not touching each other to allow for even cooking and crisping of the bacon.

6. **Bake:** Transfer the baking sheet to the preheated oven and bake for 20-25 minutes or until the bacon is crispy and the asparagus is tender. You may need to flip the spears halfway through cooking to ensure that the bacon cooks evenly on all sides.

7. **Serve:** Once done, remove the bacon-wrapped asparagus spears from the oven and transfer them to a serving platter. Serve immediately as a delicious and savory side dish alongside your favorite carnivore meal.

Enjoy the savory and satisfying flavors of bacon-wrapped asparagus spears as a perfect accompaniment to any carnivore meal!

Grilled Portobello Mushrooms

Grilled Portobello mushrooms are a hearty and flavorful addition to your carnivore diet, offering a meaty texture and rich, earthy taste.

Ingredients:

- Portobello mushrooms (cleaned and stems removed)
- Olive oil or melted butter

- Salt and pepper to taste

- Optional: minced garlic, herbs (such as thyme or rosemary)

Step by Step Instructions:

1. **Prepare the Mushrooms:** Clean the Portobello mushrooms by gently wiping them with a damp paper towel to remove any dirt or debris. Remove the stems by gently twisting them off or cutting them with a knife.

2. **Marinate (optional):** In a small bowl, prepare a simple marinade by combining olive oil or melted butter with minced garlic, herbs, salt, and pepper. Brush or drizzle the marinade over both sides of the Portobello mushrooms, ensuring they are evenly coated.

3. **Preheat the Grill:** Preheat your grill to medium-high heat, around 375-400°F (190-200°C).

4. **Grill the Mushrooms:** Once the grill is hot, place the Portobello mushrooms directly onto the grill grates, gill side down. Cook for about 4-5 minutes, or until grill marks form and the mushrooms begin to soften.

5. **Flip and Continue Cooking:** Carefully flip the mushrooms using tongs and continue grilling for an additional 4-5 minutes, or until they are tender and cooked through. The cooking time may vary depending on the size and thickness of the mushrooms.

6. **Season:** Season the grilled Portobello mushrooms with additional salt and pepper to taste, if desired.

7. **Serve:** Once done, remove the mushrooms from the grill and transfer them to a serving platter. Serve them immediately as a hearty and flavorful side dish or as a meaty main course for your carnivore meal.

Enjoy the rich, earthy flavors of grilled Portobello mushrooms as a delicious addition to your carnivore diet!

Caesar Salad with Bacon Bits

A classic Caesar salad topped with crunchy bacon bits adds a delicious twist to your carnivore meal, providing freshness and crunch.

Ingredients:

- Romaine lettuce, chopped
- Bacon slices
- Caesar salad dressing
- Optional: Parmesan cheese, croutons (for non-carnivore variations)

Step by step Instructions:

1 **Cook the Bacon:** Place the bacon slices in a cold skillet or frying pan.

Cook over medium heat, flipping occasionally, until the bacon is crispy and golden brown. Remove the bacon from the pan and place it on a paper towel-lined plate to drain excess grease. Once cooled, chop the bacon into small pieces to make bacon bits.

2 **Prepare the Salad:** In a large salad bowl, add the chopped romaine lettuce. If desired, add some Parmesan cheese shavings for extra flavor.

3 **Add the Bacon:** Sprinkle the crispy bacon bits over the romaine lettuce in the salad bowl.

4 **Dress the Salad:** Drizzle Caesar salad dressing over the salad according to your taste preferences. Toss the salad gently to ensure the lettuce is evenly coated with the dressing.

5 **Serve:** Transfer the Caesar salad with bacon bits to individual serving plates or bowls. Optionally, garnish with additional Parmesan cheese shavings if desired.

6 **Enjoy:** Serve the Caesar salad with bacon bits as a refreshing and satisfying side dish or as a light main course for your carnivore meal. The crispy bacon adds a delightful crunch and savory flavor to the classic Caesar salad, making it a delicious addition to your carnivore diet.

Note: If you're not strictly following a carnivore diet, you can also add croutons or other non-carnivore toppings to your Caesar salad for extra texture and flavor. Adjust the ingredients according to your dietary preferences.

Roasted Brussels Sprouts with Bacon

Roasted Brussels sprouts tossed with crispy bacon are a mouthwatering side dish that's both flavorful and nutritious.

Ingredients:

- Brussels sprouts, trimmed and halved
- Bacon slices, chopped into small pieces
- Olive oil
- Salt and pepper to taste

Step by Step Instructions:

1. **Preheat the Oven:** Preheat your oven to 400°F (200°C) and line a baking sheet with parchment paper or aluminum foil for easy cleanup.

2. **Prepare the Brussels Sprouts:** Wash the Brussels sprouts thoroughly and trim off the stems. Cut each sprout in half lengthwise.

3. **Cook the Bacon:** In a skillet over medium heat, cook the chopped bacon pieces until they are crispy and golden brown. Remove the bacon from the skillet and place it on a paper towel-lined plate to drain excess grease. Set aside.

4. **Roast the Brussels Sprouts:** Place the halved Brussels sprouts in a large mixing bowl.

Drizzle with olive oil and season with salt and pepper to taste. Toss the Brussels sprouts until they are evenly coated with oil and seasoning.

5. **Arrange on Baking Sheet:** Spread the seasoned Brussels sprouts in a single layer on the prepared baking sheet, ensuring they are not overcrowded. This allows them to roast evenly and become crispy.

6. **Add Bacon:** Sprinkle the cooked bacon pieces over the Brussels sprouts on the baking sheet, distributing them evenly.

7. **Roast in the Oven:** Place the baking sheet in the preheated oven and roast the Brussels sprouts for about 20-25 minutes or until they are tender on the inside and crispy on the outside. You can flip them halfway through the cooking time for even browning.

8. **Serve:** Once the Brussels sprouts are roasted to perfection, remove them from the oven and transfer them to a serving dish. Serve hot as a delicious and flavorful side dish alongside your favorite carnivore main course.

9. **Enjoy:** Enjoy the roasted Brussels sprouts with crispy bacon as a tasty and nutritious addition to your carnivore meal. The combination of tender Brussels sprouts and crispy bacon will surely tantalize your taste buds and leave you wanting more.

Broccoli with Garlic Butter

Steamed broccoli drizzled with garlic-infused butter is a simple yet delicious side dish that complements any carnivore meal.

Ingredients:

- Fresh broccoli florets
- Butter
- Garlic cloves, minced
- Salt and pepper to taste

Step by Step Instructions:

1. **Prepare the Broccoli:** Rinse the broccoli florets under cold water and pat them dry with a paper towel. Cut the broccoli into bite-sized florets, discarding any tough stems.

2. **Steam the Broccoli:** Fill a large pot with about an inch of water and place a steamer basket or insert inside. Bring the water to a boil over medium-high heat. Once boiling, add the broccoli florets to the steamer basket, cover with a lid, and steam for about 5-7 minutes or until the broccoli is tender but still crisp.

3. **Make the Garlic Butter:** While the broccoli is steaming, melt the butter in a small saucepan over medium heat. Add the minced garlic to the melted butter and sauté for 1-2 minutes, stirring frequently, until the garlic becomes fragrant and slightly golden. Remove the saucepan from the heat and set aside.

4. **Combine Broccoli and Garlic Butter:** Once the broccoli is cooked to your desired tenderness, transfer the steamed broccoli florets to a large mixing bowl. Pour the garlic-infused butter over the broccoli.

5. **Season with Salt and Pepper:** Season the broccoli with salt and pepper to taste. Toss the broccoli gently to ensure that it is evenly coated with the garlic butter and seasoning.

6. **Serve:** Transfer the garlic butter-coated broccoli to a serving dish. Serve immediately as a flavorful and nutritious side dish alongside your favorite carnivore main course.

7. **Enjoy:** Enjoy the steamed broccoli with garlic butter as a delicious and satisfying addition to your carnivore meal. The garlic-infused butter adds a burst of flavor to the tender broccoli florets, making it a perfect accompaniment to any meaty dish.

Creamed Spinach with Bacon

Creamed spinach cooked with creamy sauce and crispy bacon is a comforting and indulgent side dish that's sure to please.

Ingredients:

- 1 lb. fresh spinach leaves, washed and trimmed
- slices of bacon, chopped
- 2 cloves garlic, minced

- 1 cup heavy cream

- 1/4 cup grated Parmesan cheese

- Salt and pepper to taste

- Pinch of nutmeg (optional)

Step by Step Instructions:

1. **Cook the Bacon:** In a large skillet or frying pan, cook the chopped bacon over medium heat until it becomes crispy and browned. Remove the cooked bacon from the skillet and set it aside on a plate lined with paper towels to drain excess grease. Leave the bacon grease in the skillet.

2. **Sauté the Garlic:** In the same skillet with the bacon grease, add the minced garlic. Sauté the garlic over medium heat for 1-2 minutes until it becomes fragrant and slightly golden.

3. **Add the Spinach:** Gradually add the fresh spinach leaves to the skillet, stirring occasionally with tongs or a spatula. Cook the spinach for 3-4 minutes, or until it wilts and reduces in volume.

4. **Prepare the Cream Sauce:** Pour the heavy cream into the skillet with the wilted spinach. Stir well to combine, allowing the cream to heat through and simmer gently.

5. **Add the Parmesan Cheese:** Sprinkle the grated Parmesan cheese over the spinach and cream mixture. Stir until the cheese melts and incorporates into the sauce, thickening it slightly.

6. **Season the Creamed Spinach:** Season the creamed spinach with salt, pepper, and a pinch of nutmeg (if using), adjusting the seasoning according to your taste preferences. Stir well to distribute the seasoning evenly throughout the dish.

7. **Finish with Bacon:** Crumble the cooked bacon pieces and add them back to the skillet with the creamed spinach. Stir to distribute the bacon throughout the dish, reserving some for garnish if desired.

8. **Serve:** Transfer the creamed spinach with bacon to a serving dish or individual plates. Garnish with additional crumbled bacon if desired. Serve hot as a delicious and indulgent side dish alongside your favorite carnivore main course.

9. **Enjoy:** Enjoy the creamy and flavorful creamed spinach with bacon as a comforting and satisfying addition to your carnivore meal. The combination of creamy sauce, tender spinach, and crispy bacon creates a delightful balance of flavors and textures.

Deviled Eggs with Bacon

Deviled eggs filled with a creamy mixture and topped with crispy bacon are a delightful appetizer or side dish for carnivore-friendly gatherings.

Ingredients:

- large eggs
- slices of bacon

- 2 tablespoons mayonnaise

- 1 teaspoon Dijon mustard

- 1 teaspoon white vinegar

- Salt and pepper to taste

- Paprika, for garnish (optional)

- Chopped chives or parsley, for garnish (optional)

Step by Step Instructions:

1. **Hard-Boil the Eggs:** Place the eggs in a single layer in a saucepan and cover them with water, ensuring they are submerged by at least an inch. Bring the water to a boil over medium-high heat. Once boiling, cover the saucepan with a lid and remove it from the heat. Let the eggs sit in the hot water for 10-12 minutes.

2. **Cool and Peel the Eggs:** After the eggs have finished cooking, immediately transfer them to a bowl of ice water to cool for about 5 minutes. This helps stop the cooking process and makes peeling easier. Once cooled, carefully peel the eggs and slice them in half lengthwise. Remove the yolks and place them in a separate bowl.

3. **Cook the Bacon:** In a skillet or frying pan, cook the bacon over medium heat until it becomes crispy and browned. Remove the cooked bacon from the skillet and place it on a plate lined with paper towels to drain excess grease. Let it cool, then chop or crumble it into small pieces.

4. **Prepare the Filling:** Mash the egg yolks with a fork until they are smooth and lump-free. Add mayonnaise, Dijon mustard, white vinegar, salt, and pepper to the mashed yolks. Stir well to combine, adjusting the seasoning to taste.

5. **Fill the Egg Whites:** Spoon or pipe the yolk mixture into the hollowed-out egg white halves, dividing it evenly among them. You can use a piping bag fitted with a decorative tip for a more elegant presentation.

6. **Top with Bacon:** Sprinkle the chopped or crumbled bacon evenly over the filled deviled egg halves, pressing it gently into the yolk mixture to adhere.

7. **Garnish (Optional):** If desired, garnish the deviled eggs with a sprinkle of paprika for added color and flavor, and chopped chives or parsley for a fresh herbal touch.

8. **Chill and Serve:** Arrange the deviled eggs on a serving platter and refrigerate them for at least 30 minutes to allow the flavors to meld and the filling to set. Serve chilled as a delicious appetizer or side dish for carnivore-friendly gatherings.

9. **Enjoy:** Enjoy these creamy deviled eggs with bacon as a flavorful and satisfying addition to your carnivore meal. The combination of creamy filling and crispy bacon adds a delightful contrast of textures and flavors that's sure to please.

Bacon-Wrapped Jalapeño Poppers

Spicy jalapeño peppers stuffed with cream cheese and wrapped in crispy bacon are a flavorful and satisfying side dish or appetizer.

Ingredients:

- fresh jalapeño peppers
- ounces' cream cheese, softened
- slices of bacon, cut in half crosswise
- Toothpicks

Step by Step Instructions:

1. **Prepare the Jalapeños:** Preheat your oven to 375°F (190°C). Wash the jalapeño peppers and cut them in half lengthwise. Use a spoon to scoop out the seeds and membranes from each pepper half, creating little boats for the filling. If you prefer a milder heat, you can also remove the ribs inside the peppers.

2. **Fill the Jalapeños:** Fill each jalapeño half with softened cream cheese, using a spoon or piping bag. Make sure to fill them evenly and avoid overfilling.

3. **Wrap with Bacon:** Take a half slice of bacon and wrap it around each cream cheese-filled jalapeño half, securing it with a toothpick to hold it in place. Repeat this process until all jalapeño halves are wrapped with bacon.

4. **Bake the Poppers:** Place the bacon-wrapped jalapeño poppers on a baking sheet lined with parchment paper or aluminum foil for easy cleanup. Arrange them in a single layer, making sure they are not touching each other. Bake in the preheated oven for 20-25 minutes or until the bacon is crispy and the jalapeños are tender.

5. **Broil (Optional):** If you prefer extra crispy bacon, you can broil the jalapeño poppers for an additional 2-3 minutes after baking. Keep a close eye on them to prevent burning.

6. **Serve:** Once the bacon-wrapped jalapeño poppers are done, remove them from the oven and let them cool for a few minutes before serving. Transfer them to a serving platter and enjoy them warm as a flavorful side dish or appetizer.

7. **Enjoy:** These bacon-wrapped jalapeño poppers are spicy, creamy, and crispy all at once, making them a crowd-pleasing favorite at any gathering. Serve them alongside your favorite carnivore dishes for a deliciously satisfying meal.

Avocado Slices with Salt and Pepper

Simple yet satisfying, avocado slices sprinkled with salt and pepper add creamy texture and healthy fats to your carnivore meal.

Ingredients:

- 2 ripe avocados
- Salt, to taste
- Black pepper, to taste

Step by Step Instructions:

1. **Prepare the Avocados:** Slice the avocados in half lengthwise and remove the pits. Use a spoon to scoop out the flesh from each avocado half and place it on a cutting board.

2. **Slice the Avocados:** Lay the avocado halves flat side down on the cutting board. With a sharp knife, slice the avocado halves into thin, even slices. You can slice them lengthwise or crosswise, depending on your preference.

3. **Season with Salt and Pepper:** Arrange the avocado slices on a serving plate or platter in a single layer. Sprinkle them with salt and freshly ground black pepper, ensuring that each slice is evenly seasoned.

4. **Serve:** Once seasoned, your avocado slices are ready to serve alongside your favorite carnivore dishes. They make a delicious and nutritious addition to any meal, providing creamy texture and healthy fats.

5. **Enjoy:** Enjoy these simple avocado slices with salt and pepper as a flavorful and satisfying side dish or snack. They're perfect for adding a creamy element to your carnivore diet while providing essential nutrients and satisfying your taste buds.

These side dishes and extras offer a range of flavors and textures to complement your carnivore diet, providing variety and enjoyment in every bite. Experiment with different combinations and flavors to find your favorites, and enjoy the delicious and satisfying meals that the carnivore lifestyle has to offer!

Chapter 10

SNACKS AND TREATS

In the carnivore world, snacks and treats take on a whole new level of creativity and indulgence. From savory to salty, these snacks are designed to satisfy your cravings while staying true to your carnivore lifestyle. Get ready to elevate your snacking game with these mouthwatering options.

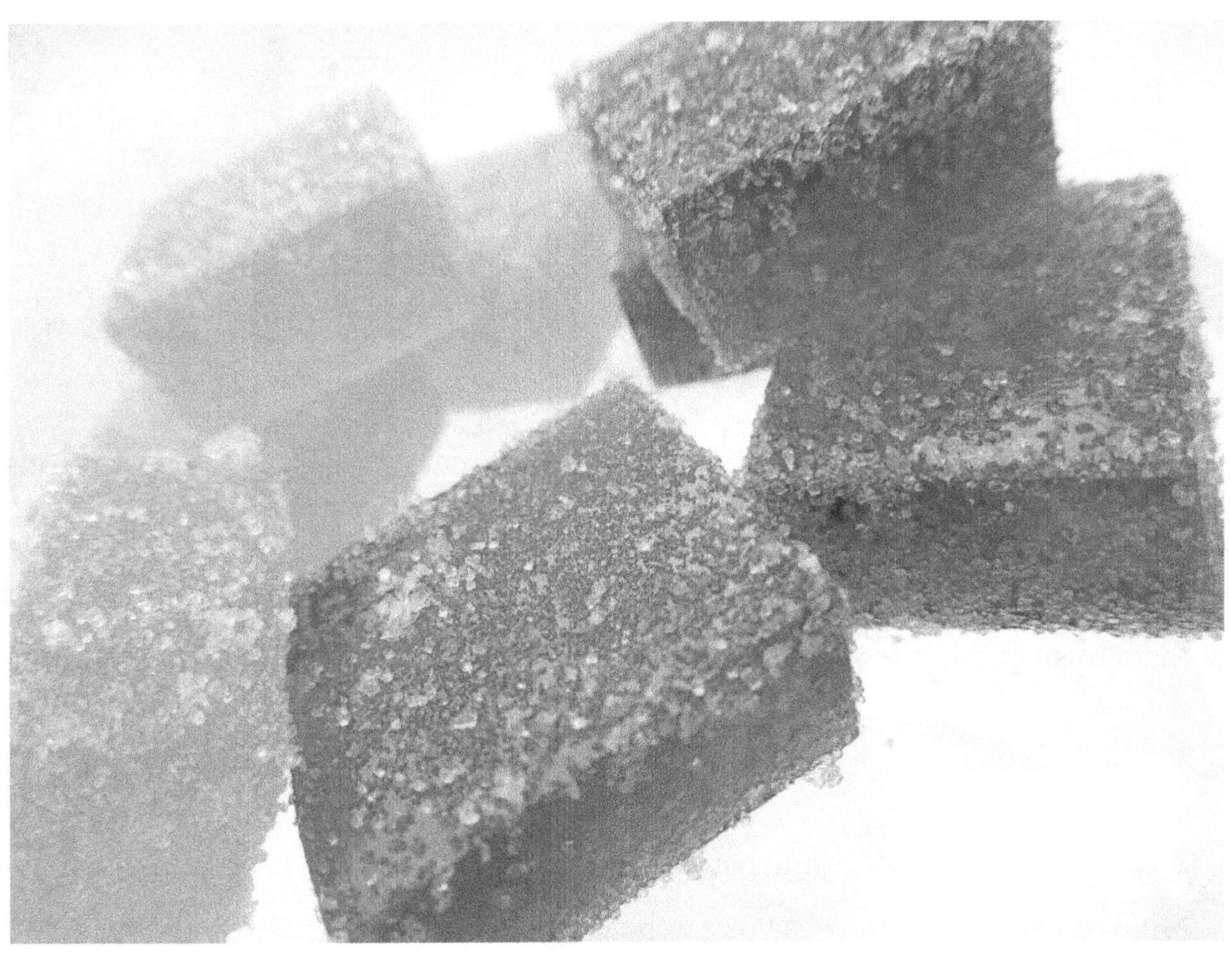

Seared Duck Liver Slices

Savor the rich and decadent flavor of seared duck liver slices, a gourmet treat that's perfect for any occasion.

Ingredients:

- Fresh duck liver slices
- Salt
- Pepper
- Olive oil or butter (for searing)

Step by Step Instructions:

1. **Prepare the Duck Liver Slices:**

- Rinse the duck liver slices under cold water and pat them dry with paper towels.

- Season the duck liver slices generously with salt and pepper on both sides. Allow them to sit at room temperature for about 10-15 minutes to absorb the seasoning.

2. **Preheat the Pan:**

- Place a large skillet or frying pan over medium-high heat and add a small amount of olive oil or butter. Allow the pan to heat up until it's hot but not smoking.

3. **Sear the Duck Liver Slices:**

- Carefully place the seasoned duck liver slices in the hot skillet, making sure not to overcrowd the pan. You may need to work in batches depending on the size of your pan.
- Let the duck liver slices sear undisturbed for about 2-3 minutes on each side, or until they develop a golden brown crust. Use tongs to flip them halfway through the cooking process.

4. **Check for Doneness:**

- Duck liver slices are best enjoyed when they are still pink and slightly pinkish-red in the center. Be careful not to overcook them, as they can become tough and lose their delicate texture.

5. **Serve and Enjoy:**

- Once the duck liver slices are seared to your desired doneness, transfer them to a serving platter. Allow them to rest for a minute before serving to allow the juices to redistribute.
- Serve the seared duck liver slices hot as a gourmet appetizer or main course, garnished with fresh herbs if desired. Enjoy the rich and decadent flavor of this gourmet treat!

Bacon-Wrapped Dates

Indulge in the sweet and savory combination of bacon-wrapped dates, offering a delightful contrast of flavors and textures.

Ingredients:

- Whole pitted dates
- Thinly sliced bacon strips (one strip per date)
- Toothpicks or small skewers

Step by Step Instructions:

1. **Preheat the Oven:**

- Preheat your oven to 375°F (190°C) and line a baking sheet with parchment paper or aluminum foil for easy cleanup.

2. **Prepare the Dates:**

- If your dates still have pits, carefully remove them to create a cavity in each date.

- Once pitted, stuff each date with a small piece of your preferred cheese (optional) for added flavor.

3. **Wrap with Bacon:**

- Take a strip of thinly sliced bacon and wrap it around each stuffed date, ensuring the bacon overlaps slightly to secure it in place.

- Secure the bacon in place by inserting a toothpick or small skewer through the center of the date. Make sure to pierce through both ends of the bacon to prevent it from unraveling during cooking.

4. **Arrange on Baking Sheet:**

- Place the bacon-wrapped dates seam side down on the prepared baking sheet, leaving a small gap between each date to allow for even cooking.

5. **Bake in the Oven:**

- Transfer the baking sheet to the preheated oven and bake the bacon-wrapped dates for 15-20 minutes, or until the bacon is crispy and golden brown.

- If desired, you can flip the dates halfway through the cooking process to ensure they cook evenly on all sides.

6. **Serve and Enjoy:**

- Once cooked to perfection, remove the bacon-wrapped dates from the oven and transfer them to a serving platter.

- Allow them to cool for a few minutes before serving to avoid any burns from the hot cheese inside.

- Serve the bacon-wrapped dates as a delicious appetizer or snack, and enjoy the irresistible combination of sweet dates and savory bacon!

Bacon-Wrapped Mozzarella Sticks

Experience the crispy goodness of bacon-wrapped mozzarella sticks, a cheesy snack that's sure to please.

Ingredients:

- Mozzarella cheese sticks (string cheese)
- Thinly sliced bacon strips (one strip per cheese stick)
- Toothpicks or small skewers

Step by Step Instructions:

1. **Preheat the Oven:**

- Preheat your oven to 400°F (200°C) and line a baking sheet with parchment paper or aluminum foil for easy cleanup.

2. **Prepare the Cheese Sticks:**
- If your mozzarella cheese sticks are not already individually wrapped, cut them into smaller pieces, about 2-3 inches long.

3. **Wrap with Bacon:**

- Take a strip of thinly sliced bacon and wrap it tightly around each piece of mozzarella cheese, ensuring the bacon overlaps slightly to secure it in place.

- Secure the bacon in place by inserting a toothpick or small skewer through the center of the cheese stick. Make sure to pierce through both ends of the bacon to prevent it from unraveling during cooking.

4. **Arrange on Baking Sheet:**

- Place the bacon-wrapped mozzarella sticks seam side down on the prepared baking sheet, leaving a small gap between each stick to allow for even cooking.

5. **Bake in the Oven:**

- Transfer the baking sheet to the preheated oven and bake the bacon-wrapped mozzarella sticks for 12-15 minutes, or until the bacon is crispy and golden brown.

- If desired, you can flip the sticks halfway through the cooking process to ensure they cook evenly on all sides.

6. **Serve and Enjoy:**

- Once cooked to perfection, remove the bacon-wrapped mozzarella sticks from the oven and transfer them to a serving platter.

- Allow them to cool for a few minutes before serving to avoid any burns from the hot cheese inside.

- Serve the bacon-wrapped mozzarella sticks as a delicious snack or appetizer, and enjoy the irresistible combination of crispy bacon and gooey cheese!

Bacon-Wrapped Halloumi Cheese

Enjoy the salty and savory goodness of bacon-wrapped halloumi cheese, offering a satisfying crunch with every bite.

Ingredients:

- Halloumi cheese, cut into rectangular pieces
- Thinly sliced bacon strips (one strip per halloumi piece)
- Toothpicks or small skewers

Step by Step Instructions:

1. **Preheat the Oven:**

- Preheat your oven to 400°F (200°C) and line a baking sheet with parchment paper or aluminum foil for easy cleanup.

2. **Prepare the Halloumi Cheese:**

- Cut the halloumi cheese into rectangular pieces, approximately 1-inch-wide and 2-3 inches long.

3. **Wrap with Bacon:**

- Take a strip of thinly sliced bacon and wrap it tightly around each piece of halloumi cheese, ensuring the bacon overlaps slightly to secure it in place.

- Secure the bacon in place by inserting a toothpick or small skewer through the center of the cheese stick. Make sure to pierce through both ends of the bacon to prevent it from unraveling during cooking.

4. **Arrange on Baking Sheet:**

- Place the bacon-wrapped halloumi cheese pieces' seam side down on the prepared baking sheet, leaving a small gap between each piece to allow for even cooking.

5. **Bake in the Oven:**

- Transfer the baking sheet to the preheated oven and bake the bacon-wrapped halloumi cheese for 10-12 minutes, or until the bacon is crispy and golden brown.

- If desired, you can flip the pieces halfway through the cooking process to ensure they cook evenly on all sides.

6. **Serve and Enjoy:**

- Once cooked to perfection, remove the bacon-wrapped halloumi cheese from the oven and transfer them to a serving platter.

- Allow them to cool for a few minutes before serving to avoid any burns from the hot cheese inside.

- Serve the bacon-wrapped halloumi cheese as a delicious snack or appetizer, and enjoy the irresistible combination of crispy bacon and salty cheese!

Bacon-Wrapped Avocado Wedges

Elevate your avocado game with bacon-wrapped avocado wedges, offering a creamy and indulgent snack that's packed with flavor.

Ingredients:

- Ripe avocados, halved and pitted
- Thinly sliced bacon strips (one strip per avocado half)
- Toothpicks or small skewers
- Salt and pepper, to taste (optional)
- Lime wedges, for serving (optional)

Step by Step Instructions:

1. **Preheat the Oven:**

- Preheat your oven to 400°F (200°C) and line a baking sheet with parchment paper or aluminum foil for easy cleanup.

2. **Prepare the Avocado:**

- Cut ripe avocados in half lengthwise and remove the pits. Use a spoon to carefully scoop out each avocado half from its skin.

3. **Slice and Wrap with Bacon:**

- Cut each bacon strip in half crosswise to create shorter strips.

- Wrap each avocado half with a piece of bacon, starting from one end and wrapping it around the avocado until fully covered. Secure the bacon in place by inserting a toothpick or small skewer through the center of the avocado and bacon, making sure to pierce through both ends of the bacon to prevent it from unraveling during cooking.

4. **Season (Optional):**

- If desired, season the bacon-wrapped avocado wedges with salt and pepper to taste.

5. **Arrange on Baking Sheet:**

- Place the bacon-wrapped avocado wedges seam side down on the prepared baking sheet, leaving a small gap between each wedge to allow for even cooking.

6. **Bake in the Oven:**

- Transfer the baking sheet to the preheated oven and bake the bacon-wrapped avocado wedges for 15-20 minutes, or until the bacon is crispy and golden brown.

7. **Serve and Enjoy:**

- Once cooked to perfection, remove the bacon-wrapped avocado wedges from the oven and allow them to cool for a few minutes before serving.

- Serve the bacon-wrapped avocado wedges as a delicious snack or appetizer, accompanied by lime wedges for an extra burst of flavor if desired.

- Enjoy the creamy and indulgent combination of avocado and crispy bacon!

Bacon-Wrapped Chicken Liver

Savor the tender and flavorful taste of bacon-wrapped chicken liver, a nutrient-dense snack that's both satisfying and delicious.

Ingredients:

- Fresh chicken livers, cleaned and trimmed
- Thinly sliced bacon strips (one strip per chicken liver)
- Toothpicks or small skewers
- Salt and pepper, to taste (optional)
- Olive oil or cooking fat of choice (optional, for greasing)

Step by Step Instructions:

1. **Prepare the Chicken Livers:**

- Rinse the fresh chicken livers under cold water and pat them dry with paper towels. Trim any excess fat or connective tissue as needed.

2. **Slice and Wrap with Bacon:**

- Cut each bacon strip in half crosswise to create shorter strips.

- Wrap each chicken liver with a piece of bacon, starting from one end and wrapping it around the liver until fully covered.

Secure the bacon in place by inserting a toothpick or small skewer through the center of the liver and bacon, making sure to pierce through both ends of the bacon to prevent it from unraveling during cooking.

3. **Season (Optional):**

- If desired, season the bacon-wrapped chicken livers with salt and pepper to taste.

4. **Preheat the Skillet:**

- Preheat a skillet or frying pan over medium heat. If desired, grease the skillet with a small amount of olive oil or cooking fat to prevent sticking.

5. **Cook the Bacon-Wrapped Chicken Livers:**

- Once the skillet is heated, carefully place the bacon-wrapped chicken livers in the skillet, seam side down. Cook for 3-4 minutes on each side, or until the bacon is crispy and the chicken livers are cooked through.

6. **Check for Doneness:**

- To ensure the chicken livers are fully cooked, pierce them with a fork or knife. They should be firm to the touch and no longer pink in the center.

7. **Serve and Enjoy:**

- Once cooked to perfection, remove the bacon-wrapped chicken livers from the skillet and transfer them to a serving platter.

- Allow the bacon-wrapped chicken livers to cool for a few minutes before serving.

- Serve as a flavorful and nutrient-dense snack or appetizer, and enjoy the tender and delicious taste of bacon-wrapped chicken livers!

Beef Jerky Trail Mix with Nuts

Fuel your carnivore cravings with beef jerky trail mix, a protein-packed snack that's perfect for on-the-go munching.

Ingredients:

- Beef jerky, thinly sliced or chopped into small pieces
- Assorted nuts (e.g., almonds, cashews, walnuts, pecans)
- Optional additions: dried fruits (e.g., cranberries, raisins), seeds (e.g., pumpkin seeds, sunflower seeds)

Step by Step Instructions:

1. **Prepare the Beef Jerky:**

- If using whole beef jerky strips, thinly slice or chop them into small, bite-sized pieces. Set aside.

2. **Select and Prepare Nuts:**

- Choose your preferred assortment of nuts and measure out the desired quantity. If the nuts are whole, you can chop them into smaller pieces if preferred.

3. Combine Ingredients:

- In a mixing bowl or large resalable bag, combine the beef jerky pieces with the assorted nuts. Add any optional additions such as dried fruits or seeds, if desired.

4. Mix Well:

- Toss or mix the ingredients together until well combined. Ensure that the beef jerky and nuts are evenly distributed throughout the trail mix.\

5. Store or Serve:

- Transfer the beef jerky trail mix to an airtight container or resalable bag for storage.

- Alternatively, divide the trail mix into individual serving-sized portions for convenient snacking on the go.

6. Enjoy:

- Enjoy the beef jerky trail mix as a protein-rich and satisfying snack whenever hunger strikes. It's perfect for hiking, road trips, or simply as a quick and nutritious bite between meals.

Pork Rind Nachos with Cheese

Indulge in the crunchy goodness of pork rind nachos topped with melted cheese, offering a satisfying snack that's low-carb and delicious.

Ingredients:

- Pork rinds (also known as pork skins or chicharrones), preferably in chip form
- Shredded cheese (cheddar, mozzarella, or a blend)
- Optional toppings: sliced jalapeños, diced tomatoes, chopped green onions, sour cream, guacamole, salsa

Step by Step Instructions:

1. **Preheat the Oven:**

- Preheat your oven to 350°F (175°C) to melt the cheese and warm the pork rinds.

2. **Prepare the Pork Rinds:**

- Arrange the pork rinds in a single layer on a baking sheet lined with parchment paper or aluminum foil. Ensure there is enough space between each pork rind to prevent them from sticking together during baking.

3. **Add Cheese and Toppings:**

- Sprinkle a generous amount of shredded cheese evenly over each pork rind. If desired, add additional toppings such as sliced jalapeños, diced tomatoes, or chopped green onions on top of the cheese.

4. **Bake in the Oven:**

- Place the baking sheet with the pork rinds and toppings in the preheated oven. Bake for 5-7 minutes, or until the cheese is melted and bubbly.

5. **Serve Hot:**

- Once the cheese is melted and bubbly, remove the baking sheet from the oven.

- Using a spatula, carefully transfer the pork rind nachos to a serving platter or individual plates.

6. **Optional Garnishes:**

- Garnish the pork rind nachos with additional toppings such as sour cream, guacamole, or salsa, if desired.

7. **Enjoy:**

- Serve the pork rind nachos immediately while hot and crispy. Enjoy this delicious and low-carb snack as a satisfying alternative to traditional nachos.

Beef Liver Chips

Experience the savory crunch of beef liver chips, a nutrient-dense snack that's both satisfying and flavorful.

Ingredients:

- Beef liver (sliced thinly)

- Salt (to taste)

- Optional seasonings: garlic powder, onion powder, paprika, black pepper

Step by Step Instructions:

1. **Preheat the Oven:**

- Preheat your oven to 200°F (95°C) to slowly dehydrate the beef liver slices.

2. **Prepare the Beef Liver:**

- Rinse the beef liver slices under cold water and pat them dry with paper towels to remove any excess moisture.

3. **Slice the Liver:**

- Using a sharp knife, slice the beef liver into thin, uniform slices. Thinner slices will result in crispier chips.

4. **Season the Liver:**

- Place the beef liver slices in a bowl and season them with salt to taste. You can also add additional seasonings such as garlic powder, onion powder, paprika, or black pepper for extra flavor.

5. **Arrange on a Baking Sheet:**

- Line a baking sheet with parchment paper or aluminum foil for easy cleanup.

Arrange the seasoned beef liver slices in a single layer on the baking sheet, making sure they are not overlapping.

6. Bake in the Oven:

- Place the baking sheet with the beef liver slices in the preheated oven.

- Bake for 2-3 hours, or until the liver slices are dehydrated and crispy. Keep an eye on them towards the end of the baking time to prevent burning.

7. Cool and Serve:

- Once the beef liver chips are crispy and golden brown, remove them from the oven and let them cool on the baking sheet for a few minutes.

8. Enjoy:

- Transfer the beef liver chips to a serving bowl and enjoy them immediately as a nutrient-dense snack. Store any leftovers in an airtight container at room temperature for up to several days.

9. Optional Dipping Sauce:

- Serve the beef liver chips with your favorite dipping sauce, such as mustard, mayonnaise, or aioli, for added flavor.

Whether you're looking for a quick bite between meals or a satisfying treat to indulge in, these carnivore-friendly snacks and treats are sure to hit the spot. Enjoy the rich flavors and satisfying textures while staying true to your carnivore lifestyle.

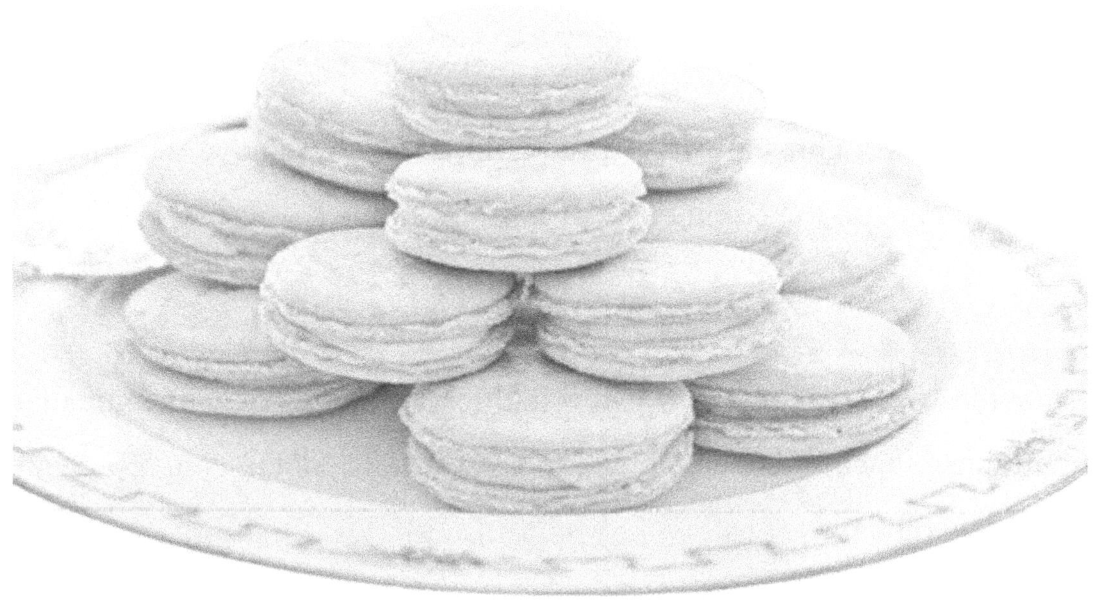

Chapter 11

BEVERAGES

Beverages on the carnivore diet aren't just about hydration; they can also provide additional nutrients and support overall well-being. From comforting bone broths to flavorful meat-based stocks, carnivore-friendly beverages offer a range of options to complement your meals and satisfy your thirst.

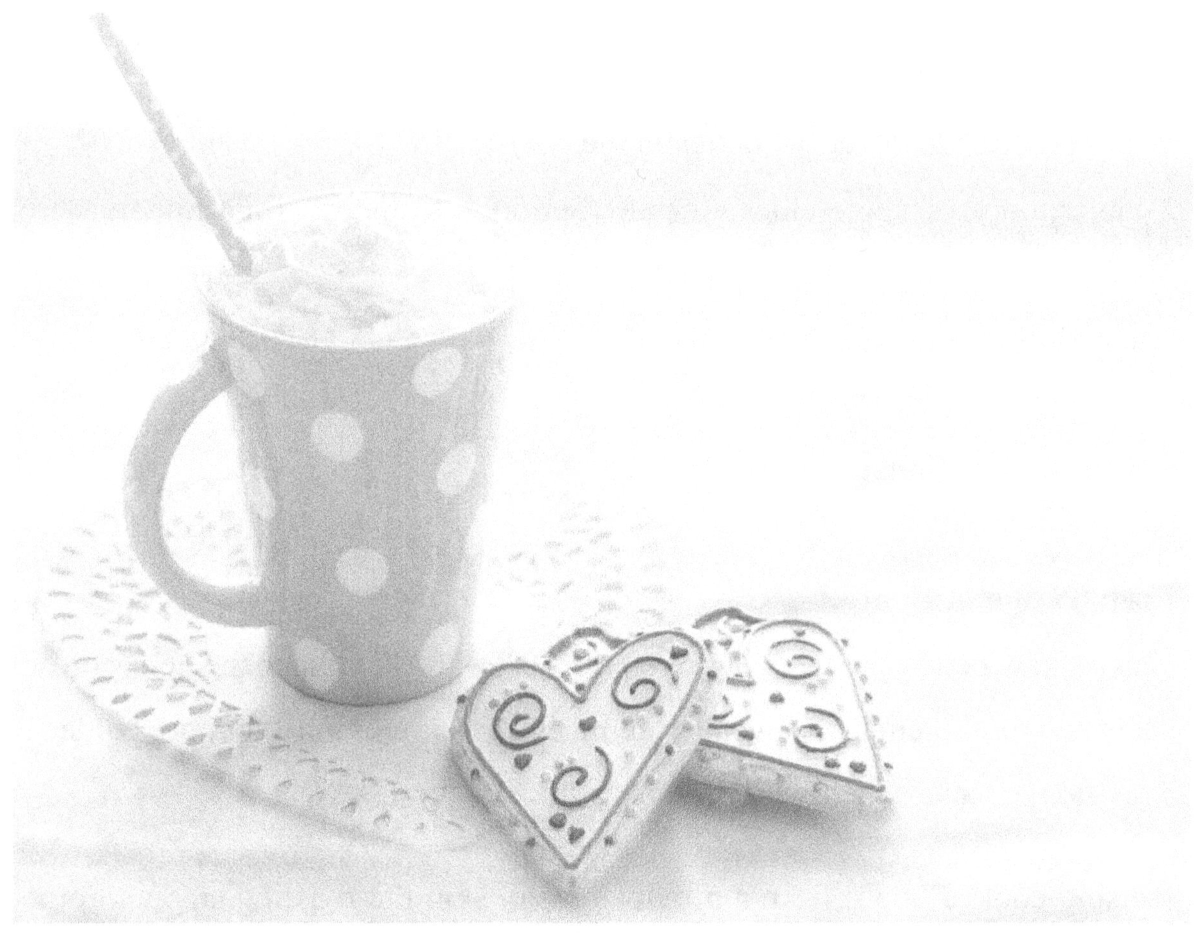

Bone Broth

Bone broth is a staple on the carnivore diet, prized for its rich flavor and nutritional benefits. Made by simmering animal bones, such as beef, chicken, or turkey, in water for an extended period, bone broth is packed with collagen, gelatin, amino acids, and minerals like calcium, magnesium, and phosphorus. Enjoy it warm as a comforting beverage or use it as a base for soups and stews.

Ingredients:

- 2-3 pounds of animal bones (beef, chicken, turkey, or a combination)
- Water (enough to cover the bones in the pot)
- 2 tablespoons of apple cider vinegar (optional, to help extract minerals from the bones)
- Salt and pepper to taste (optional)

Step by Step Instructions:

1. **Preparation of Bones:**

- If using raw bones, preheat your oven to 400°F (200°C). Place the bones on a baking sheet and roast them in the oven for about 30-45 minutes until they are golden brown. This step enhances the flavor of the broth.

- If using cooked bones from a previous meal, skip the roasting step and proceed to the next step.

2. **Simmering the Broth:**

- Place the roasted or unroasted bones in a large stockpot or slow cooker.

- Fill the pot with enough water to cover the bones completely.

- Add apple cider vinegar to the pot (optional). The vinegar helps extract minerals from the bones.

- Bring the water to a gentle boil over high heat, then reduce the heat to low to maintain a simmer.

- Skim off any foam or impurities that rise to the surface of the broth with a spoon.

- Cover the pot and let the broth simmer for at least 8 hours, up to 24-48 hours for maximum flavor and nutrition.

- The longer the simmering time, the richer and more flavorful the broth will be. Add salt and pepper to taste, if desired, during the last hour of simmering.

3. **Straining and Storing:**

- Once the broth has simmered for the desired time, remove the pot from the heat and let it cool slightly.

- Use a fine mesh strainer or cheesecloth to strain the broth into a clean container, discarding the bones and any solids.

- Let the broth cool to room temperature, then store it in the refrigerator for up to 5 days or freeze it for longer storage. It can also be stored in airtight containers or ice cube trays for easy portioning.

4. Enjoying the Broth:

- Reheat the bone broth as needed and enjoy it warm as a comforting beverage.

- Use the bone broth as a base for soups, stews, sauces, or other recipes to add depth of flavor and nutritional benefits.

- Drink bone broth regularly as part of your carnivore diet to support overall health and well-being.

Beef Broth

Beef broth is a savory and nutrient-rich beverage made from simmering beef bones, meat, and vegetables in water. It's a source of essential amino acids, minerals, and gelatin, which support gut health, joint function, and skin elasticity. Sip on beef broth throughout the day or use it as a base for sauces and gravies.

Ingredients:

- 2-3 pounds of beef bones (such as marrow bones, knuckle bones, or soup bones)
- 1 pound of beef meat (optional, for additional flavor)
- 1 onion, quartered
- 2 carrots, chopped
- 2 celery stalks, chopped
- 2 garlic cloves, smashed
- 2 bay leaves

- 1 tablespoon whole black peppercorns

- Water (enough to cover the ingredients in the pot)

- Salt to taste (optional)

Step by Step Instructions:

1. **Preparation of Bones and Meat:**

- If using raw bones and meat, preheat your oven to 400°F (200°C). Place the bones and meat on a baking sheet and roast them in the oven for about 30-45 minutes until they are golden brown. This step enhances the flavor of the broth.

- If using cooked bones and meat from a previous meal, skip the roasting step and proceed to the next step.

2. **Simmering the Broth:**

- Place the roasted or unroasted bones and meat in a large stockpot.

- Add the onion, carrots, celery, garlic cloves, bay leaves, and whole black peppercorns to the pot.

- Fill the pot with enough water to cover all the ingredients completely.

- Bring the water to a gentle boil over high heat, then reduce the heat to low to maintain a simmer.

- Skim off any foam or impurities that rise to the surface of the broth with a spoon.

- Cover the pot and let the broth simmer for at least 8 hours, up to 24-48 hours for maximum flavor and nutrition. The longer the simmering time, the richer and more flavorful the broth will be.

- Add salt to taste, if desired, during the last hour of simmering.

3. **Straining and Storing:**

- Once the broth has simmered for the desired time, remove the pot from the heat and let it cool slightly.

- Use a fine mesh strainer or cheesecloth to strain the broth into a clean container, discarding the bones, meat, and any solids.

- Let the broth cool to room temperature, then store it in the refrigerator for up to 5 days or freeze it for longer storage. It can also be stored in airtight containers or ice cube trays for easy portioning.

4. **Enjoying the Broth:**

- Reheat the beef broth as needed and enjoy it warm as a savory beverage.

- Use the beef broth as a base for soups, stews, sauces, or other recipes to add depth of flavor and nutritional benefits.

- Drink beef broth regularly as part of your carnivore diet to support overall health and well-being.

Chicken Broth

Chicken broth is a light and versatile beverage made by simmering chicken bones, meat, and aromatic vegetables in water. It's rich in protein, collagen, and essential minerals like potassium and calcium. Enjoy chicken broth as a warming drink or use it to enhance the flavor of sauces, risottos, and braises.

Ingredients:

- 2-3 pounds of chicken bones (such as carcasses, backs, or wings)
- 1 pound of chicken meat (optional, for additional flavor)
- 1 onion, quartered
- 2 carrots, chopped
- 2 celery stalks, chopped
- 2 garlic cloves, smashed
- 2 bay leaves
- 1 tablespoon whole black peppercorns
- Water (enough to cover the ingredients in the pot)
- Salt to taste (optional)

Step by Step Instructions:

1. **Preparation of Bones and Meat:**

- If using raw chicken bones and meat, preheat your oven to 400°F (200°C). Place the bones and meat on a baking sheet and roast them in the oven for about 30-45 minutes until they are golden brown. This step enhances the flavor of the broth.

- If using cooked bones and meat from a previous meal, skip the roasting step and proceed to the next step.

2. **Simmering the Broth:**

- Place the roasted or unroasted chicken bones and meat in a large stockpot.

- Add the onion, carrots, celery, garlic cloves, bay leaves, and whole black peppercorns to the pot.

- Fill the pot with enough water to cover all the ingredients completely.

- Bring the water to a gentle boil over high heat, then reduce the heat to low to maintain a simmer.

- Skim off any foam or impurities that rise to the surface of the broth with a spoon.

- Cover the pot and let the broth simmer for at least 4-6 hours, up to 24 hours for maximum flavor and nutrition. The longer the simmering time, the richer and more flavorful the broth will be.

- Add salt to taste, if desired, during the last hour of simmering.

3. **Straining and Storing:**

- Once the broth has simmered for the desired time, remove the pot from the heat and let it cool slightly.

- Use a fine mesh strainer or cheesecloth to strain the broth into a clean container, discarding the bones, meat, and any solids.

- Let the broth cool to room temperature, then store it in the refrigerator for up to 5 days or freeze it for longer storage. It can also be stored in airtight containers or ice cube trays for easy portioning.

4. Enjoying the Broth:

- Reheat the chicken broth as needed and enjoy it warm as a savory beverage.

- Use the chicken broth as a base for soups, stews, sauces, or other recipes to add depth of flavor and nutritional benefits.

- Drink chicken broth regularly as part of your carnivore diet to support overall health and well-being.

Turkey Broth

Turkey broth is similar to chicken broth but has a distinct flavor profile derived from simmering turkey bones, meat, and vegetables. It's a nourishing beverage that provides protein, collagen, and essential nutrients like zinc and selenium. Incorporate turkey broth into your daily routine as a soothing drink or use it as a base for soups and stews.

Ingredients:

- 2-3 pounds of turkey bones (such as carcasses, wings, or drumsticks)
- 1 pound of turkey meat (optional, for additional flavor)
- 1 onion, quartered
- 2 carrots, chopped
- 2 celery stalks, chopped
- 2 garlic cloves, smashed
- 2 bay leaves
- 1 tablespoon whole black peppercorns
- Water (enough to cover the ingredients in the pot)
- Salt to taste (optional)

Step by Step Instructions:

1. **Preparation of Bones and Meat:**

- If using raw turkcy bones and meat, preheat your oven to 400°F (200°C). Place the bones and meat on a baking sheet and roast them in the oven for about 30-45 minutes until they are golden brown. This step enhances the flavor of the broth.

- If using cooked bones and meat from a previous meal, skip the roasting step and proceed to the next step.

2. **Simmering the Broth:**

- Place the roasted or unroasted turkey bones and meat in a large stockpot.

- Add the onion, carrots, celery, garlic cloves, bay leaves, and whole black peppercorns to the pot.

- Fill the pot with enough water to cover all the ingredients completely.

- Bring the water to a gentle boil over high heat, then reduce the heat to low to maintain a simmer.

- Skim off any foam or impurities that rise to the surface of the broth with a spoon.

- Cover the pot and let the broth simmer for at least 4-6 hours, up to 24 hours for maximum flavor and nutrition. The longer the simmering time, the richer and more flavorful the broth will be.

- Add salt to taste, if desired, during the last hour of simmering.

3. Straining and Storing:

- Once the broth has simmered for the desired time, remove the pot from the heat and let it cool slightly.

- Use a fine mesh strainer or cheesecloth to strain the broth into a clean container, discarding the bones, meat, and any solids.

- Let the broth cool to room temperature, then store it in the refrigerator for up to 5 days or freeze it for longer storage. It can also be stored in airtight containers or ice cube trays for easy portioning.

4. Enjoying the Broth:

- Reheat the turkey broth as needed and enjoy it warm as a savory beverage.

- Use the turkey broth as a base for soups, stews, sauces, or other recipes to add depth of flavor and nutritional benefits.

- Drink turkey broth regularly as part of your carnivore diet to support overall health and well-being.

Lamb Bone Broth

Lamb bone broth offers a unique flavor and nutritional profile compared to other types of bone broth. Made from simmering lamb bones, meat, and vegetables, it's rich in amino acids, collagen, and minerals like iron and zinc. Enjoy lamb bone broth on its own or use it to add depth of flavor to sauces, braises, and risottos.

Ingredients:

- 2-3 pounds' lamb bones (such as neck bones, shanks, or ribs)
- 1-pound lamb meat (optional, for additional flavor)
- 1 onion, quartered
- 2 carrots, chopped
- 2 celery stalks, chopped
- 2 garlic cloves, smashed
- 2 bay leaves

- 1 tablespoon whole black peppercorns

- Water (enough to cover the ingredients in the pot)

- Salt to taste (optional)

Step by Step Instructions:

1. **Preparation of Bones and Meat:**

- If using raw lamb bones and meat, preheat your oven to 400°F (200°C). Place the bones and meat on a baking sheet and roast them in the oven for about 30-45 minutes until they are golden brown. This step enhances the flavor of the broth.

- If using cooked bones and meat from a previous meal, skip the roasting step and proceed to the next step.

2. **Simmering the Broth:**

- Place the roasted or unroasted lamb bones and meat in a large stockpot.

- Add the onion, carrots, celery, garlic cloves, bay leaves, and whole black peppercorns to the pot.

- Fill the pot with enough water to cover all the ingredients completely.

- Bring the water to a gentle boil over high heat, then reduce the heat to low to maintain a simmer.

- Skim off any foam or impurities that rise to the surface of the broth with a spoon.

- Cover the pot and let the broth simmer for at least 4-6 hours, up to 24 hours for maximum flavor and nutrition. The longer the simmering time, the richer and more flavorful the broth will be.

- Add salt to taste, if desired, during the last hour of simmering.

3. Straining and Storing:

- Once the broth has simmered for the desired time, remove the pot from the heat and let it cool slightly.

- Use a fine mesh strainer or cheesecloth to strain the broth into a clean container, discarding the bones, meat, and any solids.

- Let the broth cool to room temperature, then store it in the refrigerator for up to 5 days or freeze it for longer storage. It can also be stored in airtight containers or ice cube trays for easy portioning.

4. Enjoying the Broth:

- Reheat the lamb bone broth as needed and enjoy it warm as a savory beverage.

- Use the lamb bone broth as a base for soups, stews, sauces, or other recipes to add depth of flavor and nutritional benefits.

- Drink lamb bone broth regularly as part of your carnivore diet to support overall health and well-being.

Bison Bone Broth

Bison bone broth is a hearty and flavorful beverage made by simmering bison bones, meat, and vegetables in water. It's a source of protein, collagen, and essential nutrients like vitamin B12 and selenium. Sip on bison bone broth to support your overall health and well-being or use it as a base for hearty soups and stews.

Ingredients:

- 2-3 pounds' bison bones (such as neck bones, shanks, or ribs)
- 1-pound bison meat (optional, for additional flavor)
- 1 onion, quartered
- 2 carrots, chopped
- 2 celery stalks, chopped
- 2 garlic cloves, smashed
- 2 bay leaves
- 1 tablespoon whole black peppercorns
- Water (enough to cover the ingredients in the pot)
- Salt to taste (optional)

Step by Step Instructions:

1. **Preparation of Bones and Meat:**

- If using raw bison bones and meat, preheat your oven to 400°F (200°C).

Place the bones and meat on a baking sheet and roast them in the oven for about 30-45 minutes until they are golden brown. This step enhances the flavor of the broth.

- If using cooked bones and meat from a previous meal, skip the roasting step and proceed to the next step.

2. **Simmering the Broth:**

- Place the roasted or unroasted bison bones and meat in a large stockpot.

- Add the onion, carrots, celery, garlic cloves, bay leaves, and whole black peppercorns to the pot.

- Fill the pot with enough water to cover all the ingredients completely.

- Bring the water to a gentle boil over high heat, then reduce the heat to low to maintain a simmer.

- Skim off any foam or impurities that rise to the surface of the broth with a spoon.

- Cover the pot and let the broth simmer for at least 4-6 hours, up to 24 hours for maximum flavor and nutrition. The longer the simmering time, the richer and more flavorful the broth will be.

- Add salt to taste, if desired, during the last hour of simmering.

3. **Straining and Storing:**

- Once the broth has simmered for the desired time, remove the pot from the heat and let it cool slightly.

- Use a fine mesh strainer or cheesecloth to strain the broth into a clean container, discarding the bones, meat, and any solids.

- Let the broth cool to room temperature, then store it in the refrigerator for up to 5 days or freeze it for longer storage. It can also be stored in airtight containers or ice cube trays for easy portioning.

4. Enjoying the Broth:

- Reheat the bison bone broth as needed and enjoy it warm as a savory beverage.

- Use the bison bone broth as a base for soups, stews, sauces, or other recipes to add depth of flavor and nutritional benefits.

- Drink bison bone broth regularly as part of your carnivore diet to support overall health and well-being.

Incorporating these carnivore-friendly beverages into your diet can provide essential nutrients, support hydration, and add variety to your daily meals. Experiment with different flavors and enjoy the nourishing benefits they offer as part of your carnivore lifestyle.

Chapter 12

TIPS FOR SUCCESS

Congratulations on embarking on your carnivore journey! As you dive into the world of the carnivore diet, these tips will guide you through successful meal preparation, offer ingredient substitutions, help with timing and portion control, and provide strategies for overcoming cravings and challenges.

Meal Preparation Tips

1. **Batch Cooking:** Preparing meals in batches is a time-saving strategy that can streamline your carnivore diet routine. By cooking large quantities of meat at once, you can portion them out into individual servings and store them in the refrigerator or freezer. This not only saves time during busy weekdays but also ensures that you always have carnivore-friendly options readily available whenever hunger strikes. Simply reheat the pre-cooked meat when needed for a quick and convenient meal.

2. **Meal Planning:** Planning your meals ahead of time is key to maintaining a successful carnivore diet. Take some time at the beginning of each week to plan out your meals, considering a variety of meats to ensure you're getting a diverse range of nutrients. This can help you avoid making impulsive food choices and ensure that you're meeting your dietary goals. Additionally, meal planning can also save you money by preventing food waste and unnecessary trips to the grocery store.

3. **Experiment with Cooking Methods:** Embrace the versatility of cooking methods available to you on the carnivore diet. Whether you're grilling, roasting, pan-frying, or slow cooking, each method brings out unique flavors and textures in your meat. Grilling can impart a smoky flavor, while roasting can result in crispy edges and tender interiors. Pan-frying allows for quick cooking and caramelization, while slow cooking can yield melt-in-your-mouth tenderness. By experimenting with different cooking methods, you can keep your meals interesting and enjoyable while maximizing the nutritional benefits of your meats.

Ingredient Substitutions

1. **Explore Different Cuts:** One way to keep your carnivore diet interesting is by exploring different cuts of meat. While beef, chicken, and pork are common staples, don't be afraid to venture into less conventional options such as lamb, bison, or game meats like venison or elk.

   Additionally, incorporating organ meats like liver, heart, or kidney can add a nutritional boost to your meals due to their rich vitamin and mineral content. Experimenting with different cuts allows you to vary your nutrient intake and prevent culinary monotony.

2. **Spices and Herbs:** While the carnivore diet primarily revolves around animal products, you can still add depth and complexity to your dishes with the judicious use of spices and herbs. Opt for herbs like rosemary, thyme, oregano, or cilantro, and spices such as black pepper, garlic powder, cayenne pepper, or paprika.

These flavor enhancers can elevate the taste of your meats without compromising the integrity of the carnivore diet. Just be sure to choose spices and herbs without added sugars, fillers, or other non-carnivore ingredients.

3. **Timing and Portion Control:** Listen to Your Body: One of the key principles of the carnivore diet is tuning in to your body's hunger and satiety signals. Rather than rigidly adhering to specific portion sizes, learn to trust your body's natural cues for when to eat and when to stop. This intuitive approach to eating can help prevent overeating and promote a healthy relationship with food.

4. **Intermittent Fasting:** Intermittent fasting is a dietary pattern that involves cycling between periods of eating and fasting. By incorporating intermittent fasting into your carnivore lifestyle, you can give your digestive system a break between meals, which may support gut health and improve overall digestion. Experiment with different fasting windows, such as 16/8 (fasting for 16 hours, eating within an 8-hour window) or 24-hour fasts, to find what works best for your body.

5. **Hydration:** Adequate hydration is essential for overall health, and it's especially important when following a carnivore diet. While meat is naturally hydrating, it's still important to drink water throughout the day to stay properly hydrated. Drinking water before meals can also help control hunger and prevent overeating by promoting a feeling of fullness. Aim to drink at least eight glasses of water per day, and adjust your intake based on your activity level and individual needs.

Dealing with Cravings and Challenges

1. **Craving Management:** Cravings can be a common challenge when transitioning to a carnivore diet. To manage cravings, remind yourself of the health benefits and focus on enjoying a satisfying carnivore-friendly meal. Over time, as your body adjusts to the diet, cravings often diminish. If cravings persist, consider incorporating more variety into your meals or experimenting with different cooking methods to keep things interesting.

2. **Social Situations:** Social events can present challenges for carnivore eaters, especially when traditional meal options may not align with the diet. To navigate social situations successfully, communicate your dietary choices with friends and family in advance. Offer to bring a carnivore-friendly dish to share, ensuring you have options that fit your dietary preferences. Focus on enjoying the social aspects of the gathering rather than solely focusing on the food, and remember that it's okay to politely decline foods that don't align with your diet.

3. **Gradual Transition:** Transitioning to a carnivore diet can feel overwhelming for some individuals, especially if they're accustomed to a diet high in carbohydrates. If you find the transition challenging, consider taking a gradual approach. Start by reducing your intake of carbohydrates and increasing your consumption of animal products slowly over time.

This gradual transition allows your body to adapt more easily and can help mitigate potential side effects such as the "keto flu" that some individuals experience when transitioning to a low-carb diet. Additionally, focus on incorporating nutrient-dense animal foods into your meals to ensure you're meeting your nutritional needs as you make the shift to a carnivore diet.

Remember, every individual is unique, and there's no one-size-fits-all approach to the carnivore diet. Pay attention to your body's signals, make adjustments as needed, and enjoy the journey to improved health and vitality. Happy carnivoring!

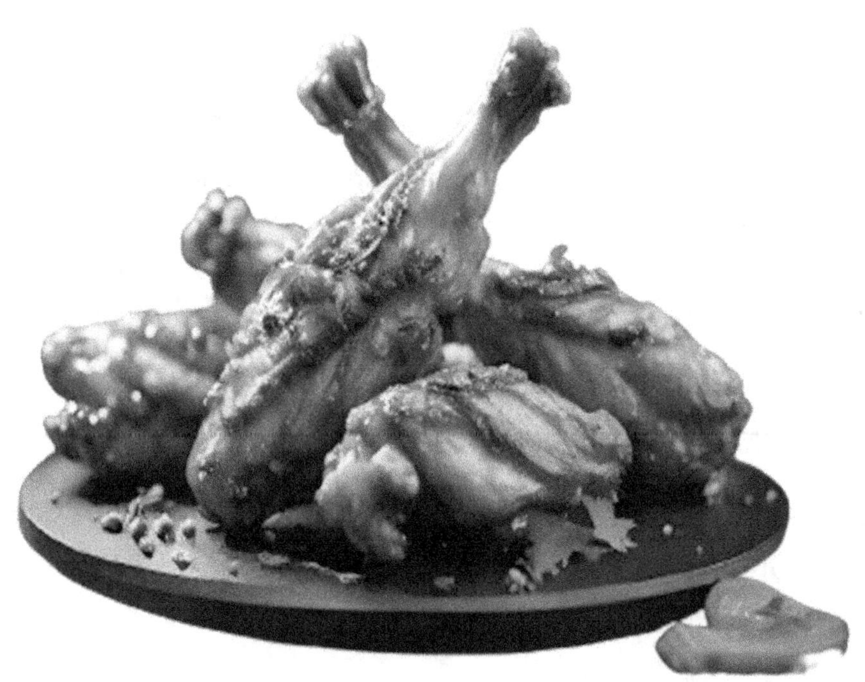

In this book, we've explored the principles, benefits, and practical aspects of the carnivore diet, aiming to provide you with the knowledge and tools necessary to embark on a successful journey toward improved health and well-being. As we conclude, let's recap some key points, offer encouragement for continued success, and provide additional resources for further exploration.

Recap of Key Points

The carnivore diet emphasizes the consumption of animal products while excluding plant-based foods.

It's based on the belief that animal foods provide essential nutrients and may offer health benefits such as improved digestion, weight management, and mental clarity.

The diet typically includes a variety of meats, including beef, poultry, pork, and fish, as well as animal-based products like eggs and dairy.

Key principles of the carnivore diet include focusing on nutrient-dense foods, listening to your body's hunger cues, and prioritizing high-quality, pasture-raised, or grass-fed animal products.

We've provided a range of recipes and meal ideas to add variety and enjoyment to your carnivore diet while addressing practical considerations such as meal preparation, ingredient substitutions, timing, and portion control.

Encouragement for Continued Success

Embarking on any dietary change can be challenging, but remember that every step you take toward improving your health is a step in the right direction. Stay committed to your goals, listen to your body, and be patient with yourself as you navigate this journey. Celebrate your successes, no matter how small, and don't be discouraged by setbacks. With consistency and perseverance, you'll continue to reap the benefits of the carnivore diet and experience improvements in your overall well-being.

Additional Resources for Further Exploration

As you continue your journey with the carnivore diet, consider exploring additional resources to deepen your understanding and support your efforts.

Look for reputable books, websites, and online communities dedicated to the carnivore lifestyle. Seek out expert advice from healthcare professionals, nutritionists, and experienced carnivore practitioners who can offer personalized guidance and support. Remember to approach new information with an open mind and always prioritize your health and well-being above all else.

In closing, we hope this book has equipped you with valuable insights, practical tips, and delicious recipes to thrive on the carnivore diet. Remember, your health is your greatest asset, and every positive choice you make contributes to your overall well-being. Embrace the journey, stay curious, and continue to prioritize your health and happiness above all else. Here's to your continued success on your carnivore journey!

Stay carnivore strong!

Patricia T. Connell

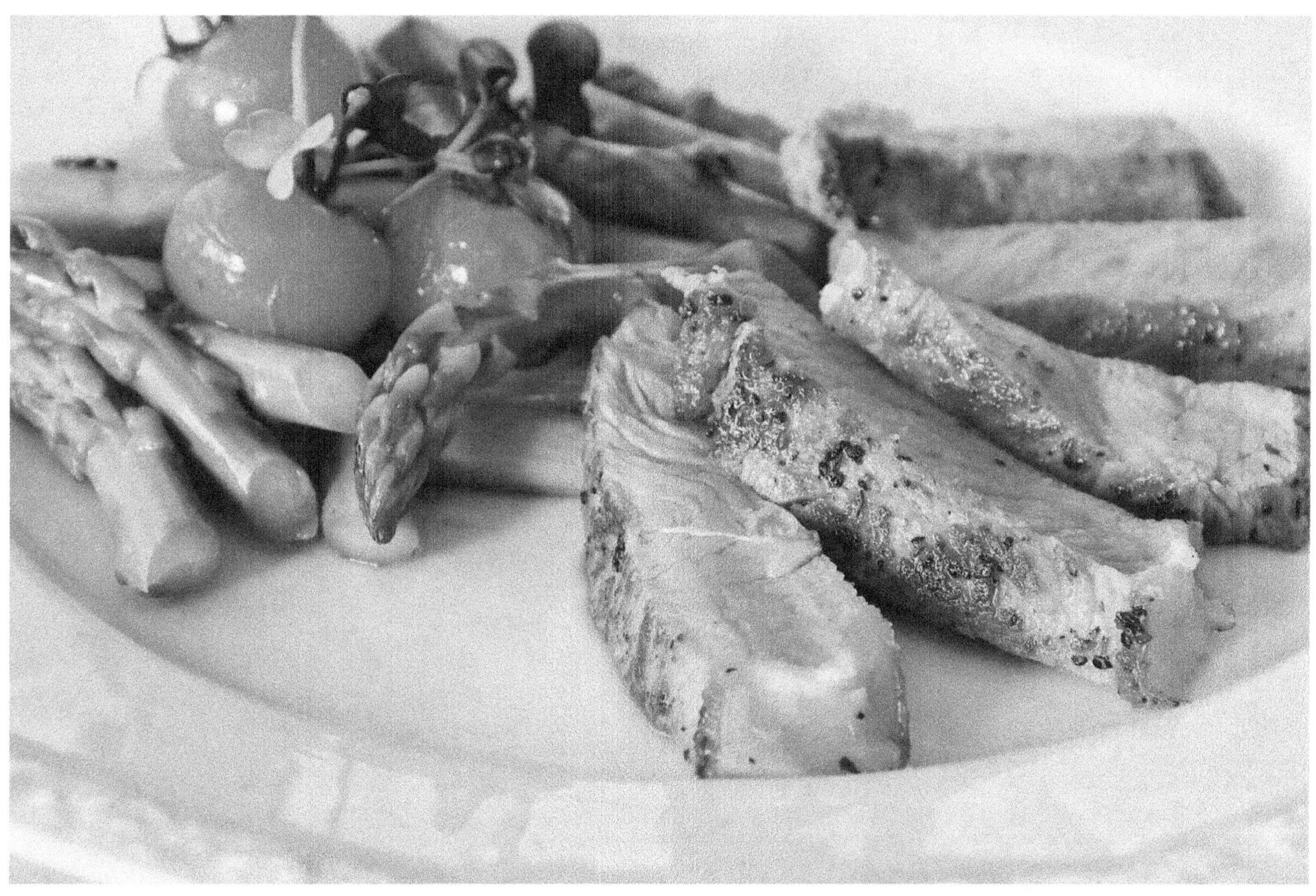

www.ingramcontent.com/pod-product-compliance
Lightning Source LLC
Chambersburg PA
CBHW080718260726
48660CB00010B/3592